LEARNING HUMAN SKILLS

By the same author:

- *Experiential Learning in Action*
- *Perceptions of AIDS Counselling: A View from Health Professionals and AIDS Counsellors*
- *Self Disclosure: A Contemporary Analysis* (with P. Morrison)
- *Women and AIDS in Rural Africa* (with G. Mwale)
- *Aspects of Forensic Psychiatric Nursing* (with P. Morrison)
- *Spirituality and Nursing Practice* (with J. Harrison)
- *Professional and Ethical Issues in Nursing: the Code of Professional Conduct* (with C. M. Chapman)
- *Counselling Skills for Health Professionals*
- *Teaching Interpersonal Skills: a Handbook of Experiential Learning for Health Professionals*
- *Nurse Education: The Way Forward* (with C. M. Chapman)
- *Nursing Research in Action: Developing Basic Skills* (with P. Morrison)
- *Coping With Stress in the Health Professions: a Practical Guide*
- *Caring and Communicating: The Interpersonal Relationship in Nursing* (with P. Morrison)
- *Caring and Communicating: Facilitators' Manual* (with P. Morrison)
- *Effective Communication Skills for Health Professionals*
- *Know Yourself! Self-Awareness Activities for Nurses*
- *Communicate! Communication Skills for Health Workers*
- *Interpersonal Skills Training: A Sourcebook of Activities for Trainers*
- *Counselling: A Guide to Practice in Nursing*
- *Writing for Health Professionals: A Manual for Writers*
- *Counselling Skills: A Sourcebook of Activities for Trainers*
- *What is Counselling?*
- *Personal Computing for Health Professionals*
- *Health Care Computing: A Survival Guide for PC Users*
- *Survival Guide for Nursing Students*
- *Critical Care Nursing* (with B. Millar)

LEARNING HUMAN SKILLS

An Experiential and Reflective Guide For Nurses and Health Care Professionals

Fourth Edition

PHILIP BURNARD
PhD MSc RMN RGN DipN Cert Ed RNT
Professor and Vice Dean
School of Nursing and Midwifery Studies
University of Wales College of Medicine
Cardiff, Wales, UK

Visiting Professor
The Royal Thai Army Nursing College, Bangkok, Thailand

BUTTERWORTH
HEINEMANN

OXFORD AUCKLAND BOSTON JOHANNESBURG MELBOURNE NEW DELHI

Butterworth-Heinemann
An imprint of Elsevier
Linacre House, Jordan Hill, Oxford OX2 8DP
225 Wildwood Avenue, Woburn, MA 01801-2041

First published 1985
Reprinted 1986, 1988
Second edition 1990
Third edition 1995
Reprinted 1997, 1999, 2000 (twice)
Fourth edition 2002

British Library Cataloguing in Publication Data
Burnard, Philip
   Learning human skills: an experiential and reflective
   guide for nurses and health care professionals. 4th ed.
   1. Nursing – Study and teaching   2. Social skills – Study and
   teaching   3. Experiential learning
   I. Title
   610.7'3'0711

ISBN 0 7506 5264 0

Transferred to digital printing in 2006.

Contents

For Sally, Aaron and Rebecca,
for Joy, Deb, Ben
and for my colleagues and friends in Thailand

Introduction

I am delighted to have been asked to prepare a fourth edition of this book. It continues, I hope, to be a practical guide to helping people in nursing. Much has changed in nursing since the first edition was published, 15 years ago. Since then, all nurse education has moved into the higher education sector and, after a prolonged and shaky start, this initiative is, I believe paying off. Partly as a result of this move, we have also seen the call for *evidence-based practice* – in my view, an important initiative. For too long, nursing was based on precedent or simply on what nurses thought that other nurses should do. Now the time has come for nurses to offer evidence of what works and what works best.

In a sense, the field of interpersonal skills has proved to be one of the hardest areas to research. There have been plenty of *theories* about how best to help people but not necessarily a great deal of evidence to back up that theory. One of the ways in which I have changed is that I have come to believe it to be important to research first and to develop theory afterwards. I also think that nurses can be 'researchers' in a more informal sense. Through developing their critical skills, they can 'try out' the interpersonal theories that are on offer and see, for themselves, what works and what does not. For one thing complicates human beings: the fact that they differ so much from each other (in some ways) and that they are not necessarily consistent. Thus, what 'works' for one person may not work for another.

While I cannot suggest how a book might be read or used, I would like to propose that it is in the spirit of critical enquiry that this book might be most useful. The contents are not all research-based (although I have included research too). What I would like it to be is a handbook that stimulates thought about how best to help. It is for the individual practitioner, educator and manager to see to what degree that is the case. Also, too, individual styles of helping vary from person to person. Some people feel at home with what is sometimes called a 'client-centred' approach to helping while others find it suits them better to be more prescriptive. I no longer think there are rules about these things. There is room, and there are appropriate times for the 'standing back' approach of the client-centred practitioner and there is room and times when a more 'information-giving' approach is helpful. Indeed, in a field such as health care, in which treatments and care are changing rapidly, the need for information remains paramount. As we shall see, various studies have highlighted the need for patients and clients to be given accurate and clear information about what is happening to them.

The thrust of this book remains the same: one of *pragmatism*, of doing 'what works' and, I think, this is in the spirit of evidence-based health care. The health care professions have not yet accumulated enough hard (or soft) evidence to 'prove' the efficacy of any one approach to helping. It remains for the practitioner and his or her colleagues to remain 'awake' to and questioning of what they do.

In the introduction to the third edition of this book, I suggested the following:

> Nurse education has become much more of a 'commercial' enterprise and we need, I think, to heed Beder's warning that
>
>> The humanistic concept of the adult learner ... is being replaced with the objectified notion of the adult learner as a consumer. According to this way of thinking, the goal of programme-development is to establish the conditions whereby the consumer, a collection of traits and preferences, rather than a person, is willing to exchange valued resources for the adult educator's 'product'. What learners learn and whether learning has any value is relatively unimportant as long as 'consumption' remains high. (Beder, 1987)
>
> It is important that this 'consumer' approach is not adopted, wholesale, by the nursing profession – although there are definite signs of its happening.

Since I wrote this, what Beder predicted has become the case. Nursing education, like most other forms of education, has become a business enterprise. The emphasis, increasingly, over the past 5 years has been on an educational system that is both rigorous and based on sound financial principles. Education, to a considerable degree, has become a commodity. Fortunately, though, there is still a place for the 'person' in all this. For, in the end, what education must be about is the person that is the nurse, the student, the patient and the teacher.

The 'person' inside the learner, inside the nurse, inside the patient and inside the educator must be respected. And it is to this end that this edition of *Learning Human Skills* is devoted.

In this edition, I have included further findings from research projects, new commentary from the literature and I have updated various sections of the text. In reading through the manuscript, I was aware, too, that I am much more tentative in this edition than in previous ones. Fifteen years ago, the field was new and it was possible to make some fairly dogmatic statements that were not always challenged. In this edition, I have tried to be more cautious and have attempted to offer *various* points of view. This, I hope, is in keeping with the fact that experiential learning has become more *diverse* in the past few years. Also, I have included a separate chapter on *reflection* as this has become an important element in a wide range of nursing courses, although it should be noted this remains a field in which further research is needed. It cannot be taken for granted that reflection automatically leads to better patient care.

Chapter 1 offers an exposition of the concept of self and discusses some of the problems associated with trying to define this personal area of human experience. Chapter 2 is an introduction to the concept of experiential learning and Chapter 3 discusses reflection as a form of experiential learning. Chapter 4 discusses the findings of a research project aimed at exploring nurse educators' and students' perceptions of experiential learning. Chapter 5 is an introduction to the second part of the book, which consists of a range of experiential learning activities. Chapter 6 relates specifically to counselling and interpersonal skills, Chapter 7 to group work.

As always, the focus is on keeping things practical. It is one thing to develop complicated theories about the nature of human experience but quite another to translate those theories into action. I remain convinced that nursing is a practical activity that provides huge amounts of personal experience for all of those who take part in it. The book remains, I hope, a practical sourcebook of ideas, references and exercises for anyone who wants to explore, further, the process of being a nurse.

Philip Burnard
Caerphilly
Mid Glamorgan

1

The Self and Self-awareness

The emphasis in nursing in recent years has been on tailoring care to meet the needs of the patient or client. If we are to understand the needs of others, we need to understand our own needs. For in exploring ourselves, we come to a clearer understanding of the differences between the person in front of us and ourselves. We learn to draw important boundaries. These boundaries are sometimes called *ego boundaries*. They represent where 'one person starts' and 'the other person finishes'. When we become very involved with another person – for instance, when we fall in love – our ego boundaries become blurred. It is difficult to know the differences between our *own* beliefs and feelings and those of our partner. When we are working with others, on a professional basis, it is important that our ego boundaries remain intact. This is not simply good professional practice: it is also survival. If we constantly blur the distinction between ourselves and others we are heading towards *burnout*: emotional exhaustion.

We all need self-awareness. It is the basic prerequisite of all skilful nursing. But why? This chapter lays out some of the reasons why all nurses need to develop self-awareness in order to enhance their nursing care. It also explores the complicated issue of what it means to talk about 'self'. On the other hand, this chapter also challenges the notion of self-awareness and proposes a move beyond it.

Philosophers and the self

What do we mean when we talk about 'the self'? Is it part of our physical make up? Is it something spiritual? Is it something separate to the body and if so, what is its *relationship* to the body? Questions like these have interested philosophers and theologians for centuries. These days psychologists tackle the problem. Arguably, the term 'self' has replaced the term 'soul'. The existential school of philosophy discussed the issue under the heading of 'ontology': the study of being. To talk of the self, in this context, is to talk of something more than just bodily existence. It is to describe the fact of being a conscious, knowing human being.

Jean-Paul Sartre, the existential philosopher, has described the notion of 'authenticity' (1956): the state of true and honest presentation of being. Sartre's novel *Nausea* (1965) was a literary description of a man's struggle to live an authentic life. He was later to acknowledge that the novel was biographical (Sartre, 1964). The authentic person, for Sartre, is one who consistently acts in accordance with their own values, wishes and feelings, making no attempt to play act or to adopt a façade. That person also recognizes the 'being' of others, and realizes that when he or she is with someone else, that other person is also a conscious, valuing, thinking, being.

Sartre illustrates the opposite of authenticity well in a vignette. He describes a young boy and girl sitting at a cafe table. They are slowly developing a relationship. Tentatively, the boy puts out his hand and affectionately holds the girl's hand. The girl, not knowing how to respond, chooses to pretend that the whole incident has not occurred and almost 'disowns' her own hand. She turns it into an object. It is as if her hand were merely an impersonal appendage. Perhaps, too, the boy turns the girl into an object by not appreciating the confusion he is causing and by not withdrawing his hand. Instead of acting authentically, both partners turn themselves and each other into objects and deny the reality of each other's being.

For Sartre, the person who is *not* authentic is acting in what he calls 'bad faith'. Such a person is refusing to be true to herself and, in turn, is deceiving others. Sartre cites the example of sitting in a restaurant and becoming aware of a waiter who is 'acting' the role of the waiter and generally 'over doing it'. Such a display is noticeable simply because we are aware that this display is not a demonstration of the 'real' person. The waiter, for Sartre, is acting in bad faith. The waiter is 'playing at' being a person.

It is possible to observe nurses and other health care professionals acting in bad faith. We have probably all seen nurses who try too hard to be 'nursey', instead, perhaps, of acting normally and naturally. Sometimes (and perhaps for historical reasons) doctors adopt a persona that is not really their own. They are 'playing the doctor'. In a previous age, when doctors had precious little hard evidence for the way in which they treated various conditions, it was probably important that they inspired in their patients a certain confidence in their ability and even of playing the 'healer'. Nowadays, patients and clients are much more clued up about what they can expect of health care provision and, arguably, medicine is a rather more exact science (although still far from being as exact as it might). Given these conditions, it seems to me to be far less important that doctors and their colleagues play the detached and apparently knowledgeable roles they once played. It is increasingly important to put forward a clear, honest and authentic presentation of self. For, in the end, all that is happening at the health care/patient interface is that one group of people is trying to help another. These days, that can be enacted in a spirit of modesty, humility and genuine concern for the wants and needs of others. There no longer needs to be a 'distance' between health care professionals and their clients. We are all people, under the skin.

The opposite of bad faith, clearly, is good faith. But the positive term does not mean, in Sartreian terms, quite what it means when we say 'she acted in good faith'. Instead, it means to be honest with ourselves and to do that which we consider to be right. Now all this opens up large questions of what it means to 'be right'. In the end, Sartre argued (along with the philosopher Kant) that we *know* what it means to act in the right way. Also, to act in the right was is to act as though our action was an acceptable one for any human being to engage in. In endorsing an action as 'right' for ourselves, we are also endorsing it for all others. For if we maintain that an action is right, it must be one that is acceptable for others to engage in. Some have argued that this is where Sartre betrayed the idea of free will. Arguably, to exercise free will is to engage in *any* sort of action: good or bad, right or wrong. Sartre seems to be saying that, in the end, we *must* undertake the right action. On the other hand, we might want to say that while Sartre acknowledges our right to engage in any action, if we want to be happy, we have also to engage in the right action. What makes us human, perhaps, is our ability to act with intention and to attempt to act in the right sort of way – both for ourselves and for others.

This was the philosopher Kant's view on how we should act. Kant (1985) said that, as a matter of duty, we should act according to what he called *categorical imperatives*. These were:

- Act as if the maxim of your action can become a universal law for all rational beings.
- Act as if the maxim of your action were to become by your will a universal act of law.
- So act as to treat humanity, whether in your own person or in that of any other, in every case, as an end, never as a mere means.

This is the 'golden rule' in philosophy: to treat others as you would like to be treated yourself. For Kant, the last point was an important one: that we should treat people as ends in themselves never as the means to achieve something. In other words, we should not treat people as inanimate 'objects' but always as thinking, feeling, sensing beings. And this is the position to which Sartre arrived in his debate about free will and existentialism, described, above. It is, perhaps, not surprising that Sartre later abandoned existentialism and wrote about Marxism – almost a polar opposite set of beliefs and theories to the individualistic, person-with-free-will position taken by existentialists. In passing, it should be noted that Carl Rogers – of whom more in the chapter on counselling skills – was considerably influenced by the philosophy of existentialism and it is worth bearing this in mind when considering his work and his approaches to helping people. Rogers was greatly affected by existentialism early in his career, and it was this philosophy that pointed him towards the person-centred approach he took to his work.

Wood (1971) suggests that authenticity consists of two related achievements, self-respect and self-enactment. He further breaks down these two concepts into the following components:

Self-respect:

- awareness of subjectivity
- awareness of freedom
- acceptance of self-responsibility

Self-enactment:

- one acts consistently
- one enacts what one believes
- one avows or owns one's actions

Thus, in demonstrating self-respect, we acknowledge our own subject-ivity: the fact that what we choose to be and how we choose to express ourselves, in the end, remain our own decisions. Linked to that is the fact of freedom: we are free, to varying degrees, to choose who we are. Finally, freedom always involves responsibility. We cannot be free and yet not responsible. To exercise freedom is to exercise responsibility.

In engaging in self-enactment, if we have a consistent sense of self, we will act both consistently and in line with what we believe. Unfortunately, I suspect, though, that we are less consistent than Wood would like us to be. It is hard, I suspect, for most of us, to be consistent in our beliefs and actions. However, whether or not we are consistent in this way, we still have to accept responsibility for our actions. Again, it is worth repeating: if we are free, we are also responsible for what we do.

Martin Buber (1958) calls the *authentic* relationship the I–Thou relation-ship: the meeting of two people who respect each other's humanity. He contrasts the I–Thou relationship with the I–It relationship. The person who adopts an I–It stance in relationship with another person does not recognize the other as a human being (with all that involves) but treats the other as an 'object'. We see examples of people becoming objects every time patients are referred to as 'the appendix in the first bed' or the 'laminectomy coming in on Thursday'. The person who is having the appendicectomy or the laminectomy has become lost behind his or her medical label.[1] In another way, we turn other people into objects every time we refer them as 'the girl with red hair' or 'the boy in the first year who has problems with sociology'. They have stopped being real people and have become known for the physical attributes or their abilities or lack of them. On the other hand, perhaps we should not become too precious about all this. I suspect that, sometimes, the use of labels is a form of shorthand; used so that others will instantly recognize about whom we are talking. It only becomes a problem once we starting *thinking* about those people more in terms of their labels than as people or when our *attitudes* towards people are affected by the use of labels. It seems likely that there are many caring people who drift into the habit of using

---

[1] At the time of writing this, I met a district nurse who referred to two groups of her clients as 'elderlies' and 'terminals'. On one occasion she remarked that it was 'the terminals who clog up the system'!

labels but are no less caring as a result. An immediate example that springs to mind is that many children's nurses refer to their discipline through the use of the – to my mind – unpleasant label of 'paeds'. There is no evidence, however, that such people treat the children, themselves, any worse as a result. The I–Thou and I–It issue is as much one of *attitude and intention* as it is one of labels and descriptors.

R.D. Laing developed these notions and wrote of the 'true' and 'false' self (Laing, 1959). The true self is the inner, private sense of self. The false self is the outer, often pretending sense of self. According to Laing, the true self often watches what the false self is doing and a sense of contempt is experienced. The false self is often compliant to the demands of others and can be artificial and insincere.

It is not difficult to see instances of this in our own lives. Imagine, for example, when we are being told off by a person in authority. What may happen is that 'on the outside' we acquiesce and agree to do as we are told whilst 'inside' we are thinking all sorts of other things. Arguably, the more 'real' side of us is the inner voice.

In Sartre's terms, the false self acts inauthentically. The person who has a strong sense of the true self, who is able to act authentically and genuinely, is deemed by Laing to have ontological security: security and strength of being. Such security can enable the person to feel able to act rather than to feel acted upon, to make decisions and to feel more autonomous. Such a person is also like to respect the autonomy and self-respect of others. This is not to be confused with selfishness or arrogance – quite the opposite. The ontologically secure person is all too aware of human frailty but, despite it, remains determined to act in a genuine and honest way. It takes courage to be this way.

We can see examples of Sartre's and Laing's ideas in nursing practice. When I was a patient in hospital, I became very aware of how some nurses adopt the 'role of the nurse' as they enter award: they suddenly become 'someone else'. It is as though they leave part of themselves behind as they go to work. They have one 'self' for their patients and another for friends and colleagues. If we notice that we are 'acting the role of the nurse' in talking with patients, rather than being ourselves, then we are acting inauthentically – we are acting in 'bad faith'. This is not a plea for lack of professionalism but just to note that there is a difference between the nurse who is open, genuine and sincere and the one who adopts a professional façade, an artificial manner and who fools no one. The nurse who begins to develop self-awareness can monitor her behaviour and note tendencies towards adopting such a veneer. On the other hand, there are times when such a veneer helps us to get through the day. If work is particularly stressful, it is sometimes easier to play a role. The point, perhaps, is that we should be able to *choose* when we do or do not adopt the role of 'the nurse' and not simply slip into in automatically. There may be times when we can afford to be more 'real' for our patients than at other times.

Appropriately, Laing was not without his critics. Sedgwick (1982), in questioning how Laing might validate his views, suggested that:

The thrust of Laingian theorizing accords so well with the loose romanticism and libertarianism implicit in a number of contemporary creeds and moods that it can easily generate support and acquire plausibility.

Sedgewick seemed to imply that Laing did not *argue* his case very well. Laing also has to be viewed in his historical context: he did much of his writing in the liberal and individualistic days of the 1960s. Sedgewick also noted the impenetrable nature of some of Laing's writings – particularly in the *Divided Self*:

> Professor Roger Brown, an experimental social psychologist from the Harvard laboratory, has remarked of *The Divided Self* that 'in the course of several years I read it three times – that is, all the pages passed my eyes but nothing happened that I would call "understanding" ...'. (Sedgwick, 1982)

He does go on to report that Brown's fourth reading led to enlightenment even to the point where Brown adopted the book as recommended reading on one of his courses. The fact remains, for me, that Laing's book is a complicated one. All this does point, however, to the fact that much of that which has been written about 'the self' can be highly abstract and that not much of it has been backed up by empirical study. The 'problem' of studying self and of doing research in this field has been interestingly summed up by Yardley and Honess (1987):

> There has been of late a re-emergence of 'self' as a focus of academic concern in the social sciences and related disciplines. Its recent history reveals only patchy interest from academics; for the most part the 'self' and its counterpart 'identity' have been virtually ignored or treated with mild derogation, particularly by psychologists, as being too mentalistic or elusive. Consequently, where there has been interest in 'self' this has predominantly existed within the narrow focus of 'self-presentation' and above all the shape of 'self-esteem'. Such work continues to be important ... but the reduction of self to the purportedly operationalizable and accessible is itself a symptom of the profound ambivalence with which researchers have viewed 'self'.

In a satirical novel, Luke Rhinehart (1971, reissued 1999), in *The Dice Man*, challenges the whole idea of having a 'self'. The hero of the novel decides to live his life according to the throw of a dice. In this way, he hopes to realize the fallacy of there being a true 'self' beneath our actions: we are, instead, able to act according to whim (or the throw of a dice). The net effect is chaos. The book also contains an excellent satire on the person-centred approach to counselling, discussed later in the present book, and should be essential reading for anyone who wants to explore ideas of the self.

Psychologists and the self

Psychologists have approached the concept of self from a variety of points of view. Some have attempted to analyse out the factors that go to make up the self rather in the way that a cook might try to discover the ingredients that have gone into a cake. Others have argued that there are certain consistent aspects of the self that determine to some extent the way in which we conduct our lives. Psychoanalytical theory, for instance, argues that early childhood experiences profoundly affect and shape the self, determining how, as adults, we react to the world about us. Child-hood experiences, in this model, lay foundations of the self that are modified through the process of growing up but which, nevertheless, stay with us throughout our lives. Such a view is 'deterministic': our present sense of self is determined by earlier life experiences.

Other psychologists acknowledge problems with reductionist theories – theories that attempt to analyse the self into parts. They prefer to view the self from a holistic or gestalt perspective. The gestalt approach argues that the whole or totality of the self is always something different to and larger than the sum of the aspects that make it up. Just as we cannot discover the true nature of a piece of music by examining the piece note by note, neither can we understand the self, completely, by analysing it into sep-arate aspects.

Erich Fromm argued that people's sense of self has become alienated because of the cut-throat, capitalistic society in which they find them-selves in the West:

> man experiences himself as a thing to be employed successfully on the market. He does not experience himself as an active agent, as the bearer of human powers. His is alienated from these powers. His aim is to sell himself success-fully on the market. His sense of self does not stem from his activities as a loving and thinking individual but from his socio-economic role … Human qualities like friendliness, courtesy, kindness, are transformed into commod-ities, into assets of the 'personality package' conducive to a higher price on the personality market. (Fromm, 1965)

Although Fromm was writing in the 1960s, he could easily have been describing Western business culture in the mid-1990s. Nursing, like many other sectors of society has been driven by a market and enterprise culture and we may be in danger of 'packaging' the self in nursing in much the way that fast-food restaurants and hotel chains have done.

Still other psychologists take the view that the sense of self is dynamic and ever-changing. There is no core or 'real' self. What we call 'self' at any given time is that moment's set of beliefs, values and ideas that colour our view of the world. George Kelly (1955) suggests the metaphor of 'goggles': we all look at the world, at ourselves and at others, through different goggles that are coloured by our beliefs, values and experiences up to that moment. As our beliefs, values and experiences change, so too do the tints of our 'goggles'. Thus, for Kelly, the person is in a constant state of flux – developing, growing and changing as she encounters life. For Kelly, we *are* what we perceive ourselves to be, or as the novelist Kurt Vonnegut put it: 'We are what we pretend to be' (Vonnegut, 1968). Kelly also noted that we *are* what *other people* perceive us to be, as well. We do not exist in isolation. What we are and who we are depends upon the other people with whom we live, work and relate. Our sense of self often depends upon the reports about us that we receive from others. In this sense, other people are telling us who we are. As nurses we rely on patients, colleagues, educators and managers offering us both positive and negative feedback. We absorb such feedback and incorporate the bits that we need to into our sense of self. Sometimes reports from others seem important: at other times they seem less necessary. In the exercises in the second part of this book, this notion of receiving feedback from others is explored as part of a self-awareness programme.

Aspects of the self

The self, then, is a complicated concept. It is worth emphasizing the word *concept*. The self is not a *thing* in the way that our livers or lungs are 'things'. The notion of self is an abstraction, a way of talking. It is a shorthand for that part of us that is concerned with thinking, feeling, valuing, evaluating and so forth. Whilst, in one sense, the mind and body are one, in another, they are different if only in that the mind is a *thing*, an object in the world, whilst the 'self' is a construct. To talk about the 'mind and body' is tricky for it is to suggest that two similar sorts of items are under discussion. The mind is clearly 'a thing', while self is an abstraction – a way of talking about something. We are not really comparing like with like when we discuss the mind and the body together. It is through conflicts like this that *reification* occurs: the tendency to treat abstractions as though they had concrete reality: to *turn a theory into a thing*. If we are not careful, we can start talking as though we *really had a self*. In fact, the self – as we have seen – is not a 'thing' at all but a suitable label for an aspect of each person.

One way of clarifying what is contained within the concept of self may be to consider the notion of *personhood*. If we can identify those basic criteria that distinguish persons from other sorts of things we may be clearer about what it means to talk about the self. Bannister and Fransella (1986) maintain that such a list of criteria for personhood will include at least the following items. It is argued that you consider yourself a person in that you:

(a) entertain a notion of your own separateness from others: you rely on the privacy of your own consciousness;
(b) entertain a notion of the integrality or completeness of your experience, so that all parts of it are relatable because you are the experiencer;
(c) entertain a notion of your own continuity over time; you possess your own biography and live in relation to it;
(d) entertain a notion of the causality of your actions; you have purposes, you intend, you accept a partial responsibility for the effects of what you do;
(e) entertain a notion of other persons by analogy with yourself; you assume a comparability of subjective experience.

These criteria bring together many of the ideas discussed above. They acknowledge the person's uniqueness and difference to others; they acknowledge the person's continuity with the past and they acknowledge the person's relatedness with other people. We do not exist in isolation: we can assume that we share the planet with other people who are, to a greater or lesser degree, like us.

There are, as always, problems with Bannister and Fransella's conception of the personhood. We might ask, for example, why *these* five factors? Do we have to engage in all of them to be human? Are we not also a person when we do not engage in the five – and so on. This merely highlights the complexity of what it is to attempt to capture the nature of the person in a simple model.

The concept of 'self' is a not a universal one. Many writers have made a distinction between *individualist cultures*, in which 'I' comes before 'we', and *collectivist cultures*, in which 'we' is more important that 'I' (for a more detailed discussion of this distinction, see McLeod, 1998). In individualist cultures such as the UK, United States and Australia, there is an accent on individuality, on the development of self-esteem and on individual decision-making. In collectivist cultures, such as those found in South East Asia, the emphasis on family ties and, to a greater or lesser degree, the subjugation of individual identity in favour of a collective identity. Arguably, in collectivist cultures, the idea of an individual 'self' is less important than is the case in individualist ones: decisions are made and problems are solved within the closer family community rather than through the mediation of people such as counsellors, found in individualist cultures. Landrine, writing of non-Western, 'sociocentric' cultures has this to say:

> 'The self' in these cultures is not an entity existing independently from the relationships and contexts in which it is interpreted ... the self is created and re-created in interactions and contexts, and exists only in and through these. (Landrine, 1992)

However, it may also be argued that, in recent years, there has been a considerable 'smoothing out' of these distinctions – especially in urban communities. It remains important to become aware of these different ways of viewing 'self' and not to assume that, throughout the world, all people value the notion of self in the same sorts of ways. These differences between notions of self are, perhaps, most important when considering the application of client-centred counselling (discussed in Chapter 6). The client-centred approach (in which the person being counselled is encouraged to identify his or her own problems and to seek his or her own solutions to them) was born out of a very individualistic country (the US) and in a period of history in which, arguably, individualism reached a peak (the 1960s). Such an approach to counselling, with its particular views of 'self', will clearly not be appropriate in all cultures at all times.

Another way of considering the concept of self is to consider *aspects* of it. Whilst, as we have noted, all the aspects tend to work together (we hope!), in harmony, they are most easily discussed as parts. John Rowan has taken something of a similar approach in his discussion of 'subpersonalities' (Rowan, 1989a), which he describes as semi-permanent, semi-autonomous regions of the personality. The analysis offered here is not an exhaustive one of all aspects of the self (as we noted above, what *individuals* call 'self' will vary from person to person). It is offered as a means of highlighting the complex and multifaceted nature of the concept of self. The aspects of self discussed here are:

1. the physical aspect
2. the spiritual aspect
3. the darker aspect
4. the social aspect
5. the sexual aspect.

It should be emphasized that these are just *some* facets of self and this is not an all-inclusive list. It might be interesting to identify what *you* consider to be the facets that are missing. In keeping with George Kelly's idea that we all construct ourselves and the world differently, it may be important to note those aspects of self that *you* hold to be important. Arguably, the facets that *you* identify will be important to you and may be the facets that you look for and study in other people too.

The physical aspect of self

The physical aspect of the self is the bodily, 'felt' sense of self: it includes the totality of our physical body. One way of considering the self is to consider that sense as being a product of the body: bodies generate 'selves'. After all, the chemistry that goes to make up our bodies is also the chemistry that produces our 'mind', that, it in turn, produces our sense of self. The physical aspect of self covers all those things such as how we feel about our bodies, our sense of body image, our appreciation of how fat or thin we are and so on. It is notable (rather painfully, sometimes) that *our own* perception of our body is not necessarily the perception that others have.

However we view the concept of self, we cannot escape from the fact that all other elements of self are contained within the physical body. It is remarkably easy to think and talk as though our 'selves' and our 'bodies' were somehow separate. It is even possible to imagine that our selves are somehow 'contained' in our bodies. It is, perhaps, more realistic to accept that our bodies are as much a part of our 'selves' as any sort of mental image we may have of who we are.

The spiritual aspect of self

Human beings seem to have an inbuilt need to invest what they do with meaning. The spiritual dimension of the person may best be described as that part that is concerned with the generation of meaning. Although the term 'spirituality' is frequently linked with 'religion' these need not necessarily be so.

Kreidler (cited by Labun, 1988), in her study of the nursing literature, found in most cases the word spirituality is often equated or used synonymously with the word religion. Peterson (1985) noted that generally religion is used to describe an organized set of beliefs and practices expressing and representing those beliefs. However, it would appear that spirituality can be defined in broader terms and refers to a complex area of human experience.

From an anthropological point of view, Geertz (1966) defined religion thus:

> Without further ado, then, a *religion* is: 1) a system of symbols which acts to 2) establish powerful, pervasive and long-lasting moods and motivations in men by 3) formulating conceptions of a general order of existence and 4) clothing these conceptions with such an aura of factuality that 5) the moods and motivations seem uniquely realistic.

Clearly, Geertz's analysis was a critical one and, following Durkheim, Weber and Freud, he saw religion as a cultural system. His framework, summarized above, allowed him to offer a detailed and broad ranging analysis of religious experience. Jung, in a different and more psychological sense, also took a broad view of the idea of religion:

> Religion appears to me to be a peculiar attitude of mind which could be formulated in accordance with the original use of the word *religio*, which means a careful consideration and observation of certain dynamic factors that are conceived as 'powers': spirits, daemons, gods, laws, ideals, or whatever name man has given to such factors in his world as he has found powerful, dangerous, or helpful enough to be taken into careful consideration, or grand, beautiful, and meaningful enough to be devoutly worshipped and loved. (Jung, 1938/1961)

It is notable that neither of these two authors necessarily saw God as a central focus of the idea of the religious. Indeed, in an earlier section of his book *Psychology and Religion* Jung summarized his definition of the concept thus:

> In speaking of religion I must make clear from the start what I mean by that term. Religion, as the Latin word denotes, is a careful and scrupulous observation of what Rudolf Otto aptly termed the *numinosum*, that is, a dynamic agency or effect not caused by an arbitrary act of will. On the contrary, it seizes and controls the human subject, who is always rather its victim than its creator. (Jung, 1938/1961)

Whilst Jung seemed to make the concept of religion 'larger' than just a question of a set of religious beliefs, it is also notable that in his definition, above, he writes of the passivity of the individual and of a religious experience 'seizing the human subject' who is 'not the creator' of the act.

Spirituality has been described as a belief that relates a person to the world, giving meaning to existence (Soeken and Carson, 1987); the central philosophy of life which guides people's conduct (Ellerhorst-Ryan 1985); a force that impels humans forward into living (Bugental and Bugental

1984); a personal quest to find meaning and purpose in life (Burkhardt and Nagai-Jacobson, 1985; Granstrom 1985); and a transcendental relationship or sense of connection with mystery, a Higher Being, God or the universe (Ellis, 1980; O'Brien, 1982). It would seem that spirituality within these definitions could refer to religion but could also include more philosophical ideas of belief and meaning in life.

Lane (1987) explains that the spiritual dimension manifests itself in four ways. *Transcending*, which is the desire to step beyond who and what people are, aspiring to be something and know something more, to love more and create more; *Connecting and belonging*, the desire to belong to someone, something, somewhere; *Giving life*, the desire to give to others, to make life better; and finally *Being free*, the desire to have and seek choices, to exercise options.

Fish and Shelly, cited by Peterson (1985), suggest that the spiritual component involves three aspects. First, it imports a sense of meaning and purpose in life, which may help to answer or tolerate lack of answers to some of the questions that accompany life experiences, e.g., 'Why is this happening to me?' Second, it provides a means of forgiveness, without which individuals may be forced to live with their imperfections and failures and which therefore provide a way to solve such questions as 'What did I do to deserve this?' Finally, it is a source of love and relatedness, perhaps the only defence against the inevitable times of aloneness and abandonment even when surrounded by others, so providing a sense of dignity and worth.

Thus, spirituality can be considered a conscious or unconscious belief that relates individuals to the world and gives meaning and definition to existence. As Granstrom (1985) notes, it is the spiritual dimension of human beings that is life-giving and integrating. It is the spirit that makes humans more than the material reality in which they are surrounded, as well as what makes humans unique from any other material being (Lane, 1987).

It may be noted, also, that spirituality may *not* involve religion. It is, of course, perfectly possible to be interested in 'meaning' and such things without, necessarily, holding to a particular set of religious beliefs. As Simone de Beauvoir pointed out, the atheist needs, perhaps, to live a *more* moral life as he or she has only him or herself to answer to and forgive. The religious person can be forgiven by a Higher Power, while the atheist has to fall back on his or her own code of conduct. In passing, too, it is worth clarifying the difference between an atheist and an agnostic. An atheist is one who actively argues against any concept of God or a Higher Power. An agnostic is one who argues that, in the lack of concrete evidence of such a Being, it is impossible to talk rationally about the topic. It remains an important fact that all religious beliefs involve what the philosopher Kierkegaard called a 'leap of faith'.

The leap of faith refers to the fact that belief in a God involves moving beyond the rational. We cannot find hard, scientific evidence for the existence of God. We have, in the end, to leap out and engage in a belief – a leap beyond the 'factual'.

It is worth noting, in passing, that not all philosophers or philosophies accept the idea of the 'leap of faith'. Wittgenstein suggested that:

> What can be said at all can be said clearly: and whereof one cannot speak thereof one must remain silent. (Wittgenstein, 1922/1961)

He was referring to those things 'beyond the physical' – or the metaphysical. Wittgenstein held that it may be impossible to say anything meaningful about that which we cannot, directly, acknowledge through the five senses. To say anything about a God would be to engage in talking about the metaphysical and, for Wittgenstein, this was impossible. But, of course, this was Kierkegaard's point: that talking of God involved a leap of faith.

The darker aspect of self

There is an aspect in all of us that tends towards the negative. Whilst it has become popular to discuss the positive aspects of the self and to theorize about Maslow's (1972) notion of self-actualization – the realization of our full potential – there seems little doubt that we also have a darker side. Jung described this darker side as The Shadow and wrote about it thus:

> Unfortunately there is no doubt that man is, as a whole, less good than he imagines himself or wants to be. Everyone carries a shadow, and the less it is embodied in the individual's conscious life, the blacker and denser it is ... (Jung, 1938/1961)

Jung suggests that if we want truly to become self-aware, we must be prepared to explore that darker side to our personalities. No easy task! Most of us would rather deny that side of ourselves or rationalize our negative thoughts and behaviour. Sometimes, however, we give ourselves away: particularly through the use of the mental mechanism known as 'projection'. With projection we label others with qualities that are our own but of which we are unaware. Often we notice the bad bits of other people whilst studiously avoiding our own bad bits. This is very evident when we begin to get judgemental and pious about other people. Whilst the shadow may not be the easiest aspect of ourselves to face, it is likely that acknowledging the darker side can help us to accept the darker side of others.

Simone Weil, a twentieth-century Catholic mystic, was both aware of her darker side and prepared to face it and even to see the positive side of it when she wrote:

> I have the germ of all possible crimes, or nearly all, within me ... The crimes horrified me, but they did not surprise me. I felt the possibility of them within myself; it was actually because I felt this possibility in myself that they filled me with such horror. This natural disposition is dangerous and very painful, but, like every variety of natural disposition, it can be put to good purpose. (Weil, 1950/1967)

Perhaps, in facing our own 'badness', we are more able to cope with that in others. We are all flawed: none of us is anything like perfect and each of us has unacceptable thoughts and feelings. Nor, according to the writer Joseph Conrad (1911), do we need to invoke 'supernatural' notions of evil and wickedness to 'explain' the darker side of the person:

> The belief in a supernatural source of evil is not necessary; men are quite capable of every wickedness.

The point, perhaps, is to face and accept them rather than to act upon our 'darker' side. Sometimes, accepting it takes the energy out of it. Also, it is interesting to note how ambivalent we are about the darker side. Certain Sunday papers offer an interestingly paradoxical approach to 'darker' behaviour: they offer detailed accounts of it, followed by round condemnation of it. It would seem that many people like to read the gory details of other people's acts and then to be reassured that such acts are very bad indeed.

It may be worth our pondering on this ambivalence in ourselves. For while most of us are horrified by what we read of other people's antisocial actions, we often find ourselves, despite it, reading on, for the details. Perhaps we are more intrigued by the darker side of human nature than we would sometimes care to admit.

We might also like to reflect on the degree to which 'evil' is a useful construct. It seems that often the term is used to convey either a sense of something outside of the usual range of human behaviour or even as an outside 'influence' on people – an influence that in some way plays on people and makes them bad. Whether or not evil 'exists' in any sense is a point worth debating. The philosopher Nietzsche took this point to the extreme when he argued that there was little value in judging people as good or bad. He claimed that as people's actions were determined by their genes, their upbringing and their past (and thus could not exercise free will) there was little value to be had in describing human actions as good or bad. He suggests that we would not describe a dog who was behaving badly as 'evil' because a dog has no responsibility or control over his actions: he is simply 'being a dog'. Similarly, claimed Nietzsche, human beings cannot be held responsible for their actions, and thus whatever they do is simply an example of 'being human'. From this point, Nietzsche dismisses 'ethics' and the idea of 'goodness and badness' completely.

We may not, perhaps, subscribe to this extreme position but we may note, in passing, the tendency we have to *judge* people for their actions and to condemn them for what we see as bad or evil behaviour. It is as though we hold it to be the case that *we* could never act in such a way. Again, it is worth looking deeper into ourselves as wondering whether or not this is true. Weil, quoted above, seems to me to be refreshingly honest in noting that she has the possibility of all actions within her. We might, perhaps, count ourselves as fortunate that we do not realize the more antisocial and 'bad' actions that may figure as thoughts inside our heads.

The social aspect of self

The social self is that aspect of the person that is shared with others. It is our presentation of self in various social situations. Consider, for example, you at work. Consider, then, you at home. Finally, consider you with your closest friend. You may well find that you are considering almost three different people! We tend to modify aspects of our presentation of self according to the people we are with and according to what we anticipate will be their expectations of us. This social self, then, is closely linked to the self-as-defined-by-others. We do not live as isolated beings. We are dependent upon others to tell us about ourselves. More than that, we *are* different for other people. Consider how the following people view you: your mother, your teacher, your partner. In each case, those people will see a different 'you' and yet they are all looking at the same person. The novelist John Steinbeck draws attention to this issue, graphically, in his novel *The Winter of Our Discontent*, when he has his hero ponder thus about his wife:

> Does anyone ever know even the outer fringe of another? What are you like in there? Mary – do you hear? Who are you in there? (Steinbeck, 1961)

Later in the novel the hero also alludes to both the problem of understanding others and to the 'assumption' that others are like us:

> No man really knows about other human beings. The best he can do is to suppose that they are like himself. (Steinbeck, 1961)

In a way, the rest of this book is about exploring the 'social' side of ourselves. For we cannot do nursing without engaging in social behaviour and we cannot engage in social behaviour without encountering ourselves.

One of the problems of thinking and writing about self-awareness is that it can lead to the idea that we are all quite different from one another. The idea of the 'uniqueness' of people has, in recent years, become a fairly central one. I think it is quite possible to turn this on its head and suggest that *we are more similar to each other than different*. In almost every dimension that I can think of, we share great similarities. We all fall in love (or do not fall in love), we all worry about ourselves, our families and our friends (or do not), we all worry about money (or do not) and so on. As we consider all the possible dimensions on which we can rate ourselves as similar to each other, it becomes more difficult to identify exactly what we might mean by a person being 'unique'.

I suspect, too, that there is a cultural dimension to this. If we read the literature on different cultures, it is easy to imagine that other people in the world live very different sorts of lives to ours and have a different sense of 'self'. It has been popular to compare people in the 'East' with people in the 'West' and to make all sorts of generalizations about differences between them. In meeting lots of people from lots of different parts of the world, I believe it is possible to see a considerable smoothing out of initially perceived differences. I suspect that the proposition, above, that we are more similar to each other than different also holds at a global level. While different people in different cultures will hold different religious views, have varying customs and ways of interacting, in the end, it is not so difficult to see the great similarities.

The sexual self

Yet another element of the self is that of sexuality. There are a few observations that may be made about this aspect. First, there is our general *orientation*. We may be heterosexual, homosexual, bisexual or possibly asexual. It is easy for people of each of these orientations to argue that their own particular one is 'natural' – as if there are 'natural' and 'unnatural' orientations. Another view would be that these orientations are simply *different*. Some, indeed, would claim that *bisexuality* is the *most* natural state of affairs and that everyone has elements of both hetero- and homosexuality within them. Otherwise (so the argument goes) we would not have close relationships with people of the same sex at all. Statistically, however, it seems more likely that people 'decide', one way or another, whether or not they are hetero- or homosexual. The point is to recognize our *own* sexual orientation and accept it. This may or may not be an easy thing to do and some commentators have even argued that it is possible to *choose* one's sexual orientation. It is worth reflecting on your own views on this issue. Do you believe that, at some point, you made a conscious decision to have the sexual orientation that you have at present? Do you believe that, if you chose, you could *change* that orientation? In other words, if you are heterosexual, do you believe that you *chose* to be so and that you could choose otherwise?

Second, there is the *importance* that we place on our sexuality. Arguably, if we are *concerned* about our sexual orientation, we are likely to spend more time thinking about it. For some, sexuality plays a major role in their lives: for others, it is simply an element like many others. There is also the *strength* of the person's sex drive to consider. Again, some people express their sexuality variously and frequently. Others find that sexuality is very much a 'take it or leave it' affair.

In some cultures, the question of sexual orientation is not a remarkable one. In some cultures, the issue leads to heated debates and anything other than heterosexuality is condemned. It is probably fair to say that in the United States, Northern Europe and Australasia the climate, increasingly, is moving towards a general acceptance of different expressions of sexual orientation. Much remains to be done, however. It is, perhaps unnerving to read the following – a therapist's view of homosexuality – written only 10 years ago:

> I am convinced that homosexuality is a genuine personality disorder and not merely a different way of life. Every one that I have known socially or as a client has been a complete mess psychologically. I think they are simply narcissistic personality disorders – see the descriptions in the DSM-III – that's what they have looked and acted like – all of them. (Garnets *et al.*, 1991)

Another view might be that it remains odd that we have 'theories' about why people 'become' homosexual or bisexual when we do not have theories about why people 'become' heterosexual. Wakeman offers the following, ironic, explanation:

What, Exactly, is Heterosexuality? And What Causes It?

What it is

Heterosexuality is a condition in which people have a driving emotional and sexual interest in members of the opposite sex. Because of the anatomical, physiological, social and cultural limitations involved, there are formidable obstacles to be overcome. However, many heterosexuals look upon this as a challenge and approach it with ingenuity and energy. Indeed it can be said that most heterosexuals are obsessed with the gratification of their curious desires.

What causes it

Hormonal imbalance? Economic conditions? Fear of death? Cultural deprivation? Pathological condition? Social conditioning? Childhood trauma? Parental problems?

Hormonal imbalance

One theory advanced is that heterosexuals have an imbalance in their sex hormones. Instead of the normal mixture of the two, they have an excess of one or a dearth of the other, resulting in an inability to enjoy full and satisfying relationships with their own sex.

Economic conditioning

Our society grants financial and other incentives for exclusively (i.e. neurotic) heterosexual coupling: from tax concessions to council houses. To be gay is expensive and many people simply cannot afford it.

Fear of death

A terror of mortality lies beneath much heterosexual coupling. Driven to perpetuate themselves at any cost, most heterosexuals are indifferent to the prospect of the world-wide famine that will result if the present population explosion continues unchecked.

Cultural deprivation

Most heterosexuals will be found to have come from a background in which an appreciation of the beauty of their own bodies has been ruthlessly suppressed. Heterosexual men in particular think themselves 'ugly', beauty being ascribed only to women. Many psychic disorders stem from this self-rejection.

Pathological condition

Many heterosexuals claim that they were just 'born that way'. Unfortunately this doesn't hold water. All human beings are the result of the interaction between their substance and their environment and heterosexuals, like the rest of us, must share the responsibility for their condition.

Social conditioning

Many unthinking heterosexuals succumb to the daily bombardment of conditioning from the mass media and live out their lives trapped in oppressive stereotypes. We should feel compassion for such people, not hostility, for their rejection of all those parts of the self that do not conform to the 'married-couple' ideal, is a measure of their loss of contact with their own unique sexuality.

Childhood trauma

A bad experience with a member of the same sex while young may cause rejection of all members of the same sex through fear. The desire continues in the subconscious and emerges as a heterosexual neurosis.

Parental problems

In most cases of compulsive heterosexual behaviour, the parents will be found to have suffered from similar difficulties.

(Wakeman, cited in Hanscombe and Humphries, 1987)

Models of the self

These, then, are aspects of the self – a few aspects amongst many. What is required now is a model that helps to bring all of these aspects into perspective. In its simplest form, the self as a totality can be seen as being made up of three areas or focuses of interest. Figure 1.1 shows these three domains: thoughts, feelings and behaviour. Each is linked with the other. By thoughts is meant the process of ideas, puzzlement, problem-solving that makes up our mental life. By feelings is meant the emotional aspects of our being: happiness, grief, love, anger, joy, etc. Behaviour refers to any action that we carry out, to the spoken word and to what is usually called non-verbal behaviour: eye contact, racial expressions, gestures, proximity to others. All three aspects of self, in this simple model of self, overlap. We cannot think without in some way feeling. Feelings lead to changes in behaviour even though these are sometimes very small changes. Try this. If someone is in the room with you now, just notice them and observe how you can tell what they are thinking or feeling. You will observe changes in eye contact, facial expression or perhaps arm or leg movements. That behaviour changes again if they notice that you are looking at them: their thinking and

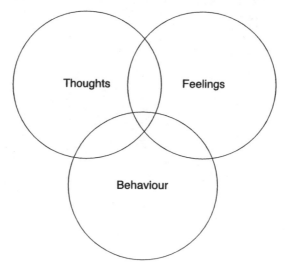

Figure 1.1   A simple model of the self

feeling changes as they become aware of you and their behaviour changes as a result. We cannot *stop* behaving any more than we can stop communicating.

This interrelatedness of thinking, feeling and behaviour is noticeable from any other starting point. If we ponder for a moment on how we are feeling, such pondering involves thinking and, in turn, a change in behaviour. Here, then, is a starting point for approaching the study of the self. We may study each of the domains and come to know something more about ourselves. As we study each domain and appreciate the connections between all three we gradually peel back the layers to a deeper understanding of who we are. The exercises in the second half of this book will focus on all three domains.

This is a simple model of the self. Figure 1.2 offers a more complex model that, whilst compatible with the first, opens up the domains and expands them. It incorporates Jung's work on the four functions of the mind: thinking, feeling, sensing and intuiting (Jung, 1978) and also an adaptation of Laing's concept of the real and false self, alluded to above. It also assimilates some of the aspects of self, referred to in the discussion so far.

The model is divided into two parts. The outer, public aspect of the self is what others see of us. The inner, public aspect is what goes on in our heads and bodies. In one way, the outer experience is what other people are most familiar with. We communicate the inner experience through the outer. Our thoughts and feelings are all communicated through this outer presentation of self. Of what does it consist?

The outer experience of the self

At the most obvious, behaviour consists of body movements: the turning of the head, the crossing of arms and legs, walking and running and so on.

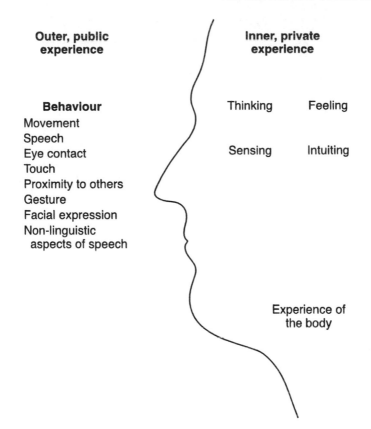

Outer, public
experience

Inner, private
experience

Behaviour
Movement
Speech
Eye contact
Touch
Proximity to others
Gesture
Facial expression
Non-linguistic
  aspects of speech

Thinking   Feeling

Sensing   Intuiting

Experience of
the body

Figure 1.2   A comprehensive model of the self

At a more subtle level the issue becomes more involved. We can note a whole variety of less obvious behaviours that convey something about the inner sense of self. First is speech. Clearly what we say, the words and phrases we use, are a potent means by which we convey thoughts and feelings to others. How we come to choose *these* particular words and phrases, however, depends on our past experiences, our education, our social position, our attitudes, values and beliefs and on the company that we are in when we use those words. Running alongside speech are the non-linguistic aspects of speech: timing, pacing, volume, minimal prompts (such as 'mm' and 'yes'), the use of silence and so on. The use of such non-linguistic aspects of speech can be a powerful way of conveying our inner selves to others. As we noted above, we are always communicating – even when we think we are not!

When we talk to others we invariably look at them. As Heron (1970) notes, there can be a wide variety in the intensity, amount and quality of eye contact. When we are embarrassed or upset, for example, we make less eye contact. When we are emotionally close to another person, our eye contact is often sustained. We can learn to become conscious of our use of what must be the most powerful aspect of communication and to monitor the amount and quality of our eye contact. We should also remain aware of the *cultural* differences that are involved here. People from cultures very different to our own use eye contact in other ways. It is important that we do not interpret such different use of eye contact inappropriately.

Touch in relation to others is another important aspect of our outer experience. Typically, in this culture, we touch more those people to whom we are close: members of the family, lovers and very close friends. Nursing involves a high degree of this personal aspect of human interaction and it is important that, as with eye contact, we learn to monitor and consciously use the facility of touch. It is worth noting, too, that some people are 'high touchers' and others 'low touchers'. Some people like being touched and like touching others; other people are repelled by it. Also, all touching should be unambiguous: clearly touch has sexual connotations for some people.

When we communicate orally with others, we tend to stand or sit close to them. How near we stand or sit in relation to others is determined by a number of factors – the level of intimacy we have with them, our relationship with them and whether or not we are dominant or submissive in that relationship (Brown, 1965). In the nursing profession, nurses tend to be in a dominant position *vis-à-vis* their patients and will tend to stand closer to their patients than would be the case in ordinary day-to-day relationships. It is useful to imagine that we are surrounded by an invisible bubble, the threshold of which can only be crossed by certain other people. If people accidentally break through the bubble and touch us, they tend to withdraw quickly to avoid embarrassment to both parties. The issue of proximity to others needs close consideration. We need to become aware of how close or distant we like to be in relation to others. We need also to note other people's preferences and to be sensitive towards them. One useful way of judging this distance between you and the other person is to allow the other person to set that distance. In other words, you invite the other person to draw up a chair or you allow them to determine where *they* will stand in relation to you and not vice versa. Once again, as we become more self-aware, so we gain more insight into the needs and wants of others.

One of the clearest indicators of our inner experience is facial expression. Frowns and smiles do much to convey the feelings that are being experienced inside. It is important that facial expression and speech are congruent or matched. We have all experienced the person who *says* that they are cheerful or upset but whose facial expression suggests otherwise. Bandler and Grinder (1975) note that for the purposes of clear communication, three aspects of our outer behaviour must match: general body position, content of speech and facial expression. If two or more of these are mismatched then our communication will be confused and confusing. Thus if we *say* that we are cheerful but shrug our shoulders and have an unhappy expression, the message will be unclear. We can do a lot to improve our communication on this level. It is insufficient just to *say* what we mean. We must be *seen* to mean it as well.

Two issues become clear from this brief analysis of the outer aspects of self. We can become aware of our use of speech, eye contact, touch, proximity to others, gesture, facial expression and non-linguistic aspects of speech as a means of deepening our understanding of ourselves. Also, by becoming conscious of how we use those verbal and non-verbal behaviours we can use them more skilfully to enhance our contact with others. We can increase our interpersonal skills by intentionally using ourselves as instruments. Heron uses the expression 'conscious use of self' (Heron, 1973) to convey this concept. This is not to say that we need to become robotic and artificial but to note that in caring for others we can more precisely use our 'selves' as instruments of communication.

The inner experience of the self

The inner, private experience in this model may be divided into four aspects of mental functioning – thinking, feeling, sensing and intuiting – and the experience of the body. Clearly, the division of these aspects into two groups is artificial as both mental and physical events are inter-related. As Searle (1983) points out, a mental event is also a physical event. To think that it is not is to perpetuate the old philosophical problem of mind/body dualism. This is sometimes know as Cartesian dualism after the philosopher René Descartes, who believed that mental and physical events could be considered separately. Today, the tendency is towards healing this split and interest continues to develop in concepts of holistic nursing and holistic medicine – both of which treat the mind and body together. As we have already noted, any concept of the self must take into account the mind and the body as a totality. On the other hand, it is important to note that sometimes it is useful to consider the body and mind separately. From the point of view of clarifying what we mean by 'mind', for example and from the point of view of learning physiology. It has become something of an easy-to-state cliché that 'the mind and the body cannot be separated'. We need to know exactly what we mean when we use this expression.

The thinking dimension

In this model, thinking refers to all the aspects, logical and otherwise, of our mental processes. One moment's reflection on thinking will reveal that it is not a linear process. We do not think in sentences or even in a series of phrases. The process is much more haphazard than that. The technique known as 'free-association' and used in psychoanalysis demonstrates the apparently random nature of some of our thinking. Free association demands the individual verbalizes whatever comes into his or her mind, without any attempt at censoring or of stopping the flow. Try to do this. The process is always difficult and sometimes impossible. The reasons for this are outlined in the psychoanalytical literature and such theory can offer insights into the genesis and nature of thought processes.

Clearly, not everybody wants or can afford psychoanalysis but its ideas can be useful in attempting to understand thinking.

Arguably, the domain of thinking is more dominant in certain individuals. Certainly, thinking is highly rated in our culture and the education system sometimes seems to concern itself *only* with this mode. The domains of feeling, sensing and intuiting are usually less well catered for. In nursing, however, we are concerned with all sorts of feelings, from pain to anxiety, from depression to elation. Understanding these requires the use of dimensions other than thinking. On the other hand, it is obviously important that we all develop the thinking aspect. If we are to progress as a research-based profession and if we are to be able to demonstrate critical awareness, we must be able to think clearly. We must also be able to appreciate when feeling gets in the way of thinking, as well as vice versa.

The feeling dimension

Feeling in this model refers to the emotional aspect of the person: love, sadness, joy, happiness etc. Heron (1977a) argues that there are four dominant aspects of emotion that are frequently denied and repressed in our culture: anger, grief, fear and embarrassment. He argues that anger can be expressed through loud sound and shouting, grief through tears, fear through trembling and embarrassment through laughter. He argues, further, that such expression of emotion (or catharsis) is a healthy process. Heron claims that we live in a non-cathartic culture and the general tendency is to encourage people to control rather than to express emotion. As a result, we all carry round with us a pool of un-expressed emotion that distorts our thinking and stops us functioning fully. If we can learn to express some of this bottled-up emotion – and methods of doing this will be discussed later – then we can become more open to experience, less fearful and anxious and we can exercise more self-determination and autonomy. Part of becoming self-aware entails discovering and exploring the emotional dimension.

Nurses must deal with other people's emotions and there may be a link between the way in which we handle our own emotions and the way in which we handle those of others. If we understand and can appropriately express our own anger, fear, grief and embarrassment, we will be better able to handle them in other people. In caring for others, we must get to know ourselves better.

Certainly other people's emotions affect us and stir up our own, un-expressed emotions. Try this simple experiment. Next time a programme on television moves you near to tears, turn off the set and allow yourself to cry. As you do so, reflect on what it is you are crying about. It is highly likely that the issue causing the tears is a personal one, not directly related to the television programme. Most people carry around with them this unexpressed emotion, just beneath the surface. Nurses who work in particularly emotionally charged environments – children's wards, intensive therapy units, psychiatric units and so forth – may want to consider self-help methods for exploring their own hidden emotions. Co-counselling, discussed in the next chapter, is one such method and others are discussed by Bond (1986) and Bond and Kilty (1982). Alternatively, consider going to the cinema as a means of emotional release ... what do most people go to the cinema for? To cry, to allow themselves to get frightened, or to laugh. The cinema, and to a lesser extent, the theatre, concerts and sporting events, offer 'natural' release valves for people's pent up emotion.

The sensing dimension

The sensing dimension in the model refers to inputs through the five special senses – touch, taste, smell, hearing, sight – and also to proprioceptive and kinaesthetic sense. Proprioception refers to our ability to know the position of our bodies and thus to know where we are in space. We do not, for instance, need to *think* about our body position most of the time. We are fed that information by bundles of nerve fibres known as proprioceptors. Kinaesthetic sense refers to our sense of body movement. Again, this is not a sense that we normally have to think about.

We can make ourselves aware of any of the senses. Another simple experiment will demonstrate this. Stop reading for a moment and pay attention to everything that you can hear. Take in all the sounds around you: the more subtle as well as the more obvious. In doing so, notice how much of this one particular sense is normally passed over and how many sounds are usually filtered out of consciousness. At times it is vital that our senses are selective and that extraneous sounds, images, smells and so on are banished from awareness. On the other hand, often that filtering mechanism becomes *too* efficient and we filter out or fail to notice many sounds and sights that are around us all the time. We live half asleep.

In developing an awareness of our senses, we can begin to notice the world again. Just as importantly, we can begin to notice *each other* again. In developing our sense of sight, for instance, we can begin to notice subtle changes in other people's expressions, body postures and other aspects of non-verbal communication. Without that awareness we may miss a considerable amount of essential interpersonal information. In nursing, the value of such awareness is clear. Nurses need to be observant. What is not always so clear is *how* nurses are supposed to become observant. Like any other skills development, training to notice takes time and practice. The redeeming feature is that it is a skill that *individuals* can develop for themselves. In a way, it is simply a matter of *remembering* to notice. Eventually, such awareness or 'staying awake' becomes part of the person.

The intuitive dimension

The intuitive dimension is perhaps the most undervalued. Intuition refers to knowledge and insight that arrives independently of the senses. In other words we just 'know'. Ornstein (1975), who studies the literature on the differences between the two sides of the brain, identified intuition with the right side. He argued that the two sides have qualitatively different functions. The left side is concerned with cognitive processes and with rationality. The right is more to do with holism, creativity and intuition, according to Ornstein. If he is right, the implication is that if the intuitive aspect is developed further (along with creativity) then both sides of the brain will function optimally. Ornstein argues that the present Western culture is dominated by the left brain approach to education and development. He calls for an educational system that honours creativity and intuition *alongside* the development of rationality.

Perhaps we neglect intuition through fear of it or concern that it may not be trusted. On the other hand, it is likely that we all have 'hunches' that when followed turn out to be 'right'. Many aspects of nursing require the nurse to be intuitive. Sometimes, in order to empathize with another person we have to guess at what they are feeling. Sometimes we seem to 'know' what they are feeling. Certainly, group work and counselling depend to a fair degree on this intuitive ability. Carl Rogers, founder of client-centred counselling, noted that when he had a hunch about something that was happening in a counselling session it invariably helped if he verbalized that intuition (Rogers, 1967). Using intuition consciously and openly takes courage and sometimes it is wrong. On the other hand, used hand in hand with more traditional forms of thinking, it can enhance the nurse–patient relationship in a way that logic, on its own, never can.

It is worth considering the *nature* of intuition. Where does it come from? *How* do we intuit? One argument is that intuition is simply a type of 'mental shorthand'. When we do not know something very well, we have to go through fairly complicated and structured mental processes in order to recall it. Consider, for example, how most people remember the names of the *cranial nerves*: they have to use a mnemonic or 'remembering device'. First, they recall the mnemonic, then the mnemonic helps them to recall the names of the *cranial nerves*. On the other hand, with something we know very well, the process is different. We do not have to go through all the stages of 'remembering' – we simply dive straight in at the thing we want to recall. An example of this sort of remembering is driving a car. When we drive, we do not go through all the stages of remembering how to put in the clutch or how to use the brakes. We simply do the necessary things that make these things work. So may it be with intuition. Perhaps we no longer have to go through all the 'stages of thinking' but come up with answers very quickly.

The experience of the body

The third aspect of the model of self-awareness is the experience of the body. If the mind and body are directly interrelated, perhaps inseparable, then any mental activity will affect the body and vice versa. It is notable, however, that much of the literature in nursing and medicine divides the person into separate psychological and physiological entities. Indeed, the two spheres are treated, typically, by different practitioners: general nurses care for physical ailments and psychiatric nurses for psychological problems. All this may change with the implementation of the guidelines in Project 2000 that may help to marry the two aspects of self back together via nurses' studying the whole person.

It is easy to talk as though the mind and body were separate. Indeed, we do not *have* a mind/body, we *are* our mind/body. Everything that we refer to as being part of our mind and body is part of our selves. Expressions such as 'I'm not happy with my body' or 'I've got that sort of mind' indicate how easy it is for us to dissociate ourselves from either the body or the mind.

Coming to notice body feelings takes time and patience. Of course, appreciation of inner bodily experiences is limited to some degree by the supply of sensory nerve endings to certain aspects of the body. Some parts are better served than others. On the other hand, it is easy to lose touch with those bodily sensations of which we *may* become aware. Before you read any further, just take a moment to notice what is going on inside your body. What do you notice? Are there areas of muscle tension? Are the muscles of your stomach pulled in tightly? Can you become aware of your breathing? Are you breathing deeply into your stomach or is your breathing light and shallow? What happens when you make small changes to your body? What happens when you relax sets of muscles or change your breathing?

All of the information that can be gleaned from the body can enable us to appreciate something about our psychological status. Tension in sets of muscles, for example, may be the first we know of the fact that we are anxious or tense. Learning to 'listen' to the body in this way can help us to more accurately assess our true feelings about ourselves and others. Wilhelm Reich (1949), a psychoanalyst who was particularly interested in the mind/body relationship, advanced the notion of 'character armour'. Reich maintained that our emotional feelings could become trapped within sets of muscles and consequently affected posture and movement. He suggested that direct manipulation of those sets of muscles could release the emotion trapped within them with characteristic emotional release of catharsis. Such work on the body has become known as Reichian bodywork (Totton and Edmonston, 1984) and can be a powerful and effective means of developing self-awareness through direct body contact.

Similar but different methods of this sort that involve direct physical contact include Rolfing (Rolf, 1973), bioenergetics (Lowen, 1967) and Feldenkrais (Feldenkrais, 1972), three bodywork methods that have developed out of Reich's original formulation. Less dramatic but valid methods of body/mind exploration include massage, yoga, the martial arts, certain types of meditation, the Alexander technique (Alexander, 1969), dance and certain types of sport. Examples of meditative techniques are included in Chapter 7 of this book.

All these methods can enhance awareness of self through attention to changes in the body and thus create insight into psychological states. They can also aid the development of awareness of body image. Observations of people in everyday life will reveal how frequently people walk around with lop-sided shoulders, a stooping gait or even with either side of their face showing different expressions. Often, too, they seem to be totally unaware of these things. Bodywork methods can enable the individual to develop greater physical symmetry and balance, better posture, improved breathing and a healthier physical status, generally. All aspects of nursing call for psychological and physical stamina and are taxing on the mind/body. These methods in combination with more traditional approaches to self-awareness can lead to a powerful and healthy approach to self-care. Perhaps burnout, so frequently a problem of occupations that depend upon a high degree of human contact, can be prevented effectively through this mix of attention to the body and mind.

Self-awareness

Through my self-disclosure, I let others know my soul. They can know it, really know it, only as I make it known. I am beginning to suspect that I can't even know my soul except as I disclose it. I suspect that I will know myself for real at the exact moment that I have succeeded in making it known through my disclosure to another person. (Jourard, 1964)

A model of the self has been outlined which takes account of the inner and outer aspects of the concept and which has attempted to marry the mind and body. The question now arises: what is self-awareness?

A first point that needs to be made is that what is not being discussed is 'self-consciousness', in the everyday sense of the word. To be self-conscious is to be embarrassed by ourselves, to be painfully aware of our being observed by others. Sartre (1956) describes this well when he suggests that under the scrutinizing gaze of the other person, we are turned into an object, a 'thing'. It is our response to being treated in this way that causes us to become self-conscious. For the very self-conscious person, this sense of being treated as an object is exaggerated by that person him or herself. In being too acutely aware of other people's attention, they imagine themselves to be more acutely scrutinized than is actually the case. It is rather like having someone watch us undertaking a skill such as giving an injection. We tend to (a) become deskilled by their watching us and (b) imagine that they are being highly critical. Self-consciousness is a bit like this. It tends to make you awkward and tends to make you feel criticized. This is true, for example, of the adolescent who imagines (usually falsely) that they are being looked at with highly critical eyes. Their own sense of insecurity is projected onto the world and they imagine that others view them as harshly and as critically as they view themselves.

Clearly, such self-consciousness is more of a hindrance than a help when it comes to relating to others, as any acutely shy person knows. Yet such self-consciousness is far removed from self-awareness and may indicate a false or exaggerated self-concept.

Self-awareness refers to the gradual and continuous process of noticing and exploring aspects of the self, whether behavioural, psychological or physical, with the intention of developing personal and interpersonal understanding. Such awareness is probably best not developed for its own sake: it is intimately bound up with our relationships with others. To become more aware of and to have a deeper understanding of ourselves is to have a sharper and clearer picture of what is happening to others. In this sense, it is a process of discrimination. The more that we can discriminate ourselves from others, the more we can understand our similarities. If we are unaware and blind to our own selves then we are likely to remain blind to others. A rather crude illustration may help to drive this point home. If I buy a red sweater, I immediately notice how many other people are wearing red sweaters – a fact of which I was not aware before the purchase. In noticing that fact about others I can also notice other things about them. And so, if I let it, the process escalates. I can notice more subtle differences between persons but also their similarities. The point is that the process begins with me. I must first examine myself.

Such a process of examination requires patience and honesty. It is easy to fall into the trap of *interpreting* thoughts, feelings and behaviour, rather than (initially at least) merely noticing them. That interpretation logically comes *after* we have gathered the data, after we have clearly described to ourselves our present status. This stage of self-awareness training may be likened to the assessment stage of the nursing process. Information about the self is gathered in order to develop a clearer picture, before any attempt is made to problem-solve, decide upon changes, or identify reasons for the way we are.

This approach may be described as a phenomenological one (Spinelli, 1989). Phenomenology is a branch of philosophy that is concerned with attempting to *describe* things as they appear to be without recourse to making value-judgements about them. Thus, in the human context, a phenomenological approach to self-awareness training would concern itself purely with *describing* aspects of the self as they surface and become known. Such an approach demands that we suspend judgement on ourselves. Instead of telling ourselves that 'this bit of me is O.K. . . . . this bit is bad and needs to be changed', we merely note that it *is as it is*. Once we have more data at our disposal, the answer to the question 'why?' may become self-evident. To jump to hasty conclusions may be either (a) to be harshly critical of ourselves or (b) to wreck the project altogether because we are disenchanted. Certainly, the road to self-awareness is not an easy one to tread, but the phenomenological approach can make it bearable. After all, if *we* don't accept ourselves, who will? If we don't accept ourselves, will we accept other people?

This method of description rather than interpretation is of great value in group settings and in counselling. When experiential learning is discussed in the next chapter, the notion of the phenomenological role of the facilitator is described. In this role, the facilitator of the group does not attempt to offer interpretations of what is happening in the group but limits him or herself to descriptions of events and of behaviours and encourages other group members to do the same. In the context of counselling, the phenomenological approach also pays dividends. If we can stand back and avoid interpreting what it is we think our clients are saying, we give them the chance to make *their own* interpretations. This attitude towards counselling is known as the client-centred approach (Rogers, 1967; Burnard, 1989a) and is discussed, in more detail, later in this book. It is argued that the only person who *can* make a valid interpretation of their own behaviour is the individual himself.

Abraham Maslow offered another view of self-awareness with his notion of 'self-actualization' of the ability to develop to the full those potentialities that, Maslow would argue, are contained within all of us:

> healthy individuals find it possible to accept themselves and their own nature without chagrin or complaint or, for that matter, even without thinking about the matter very much. They can accept their own human nature with all its discrepancies from the ideal image without feeling real concern. It would convey the wrong impression to say that they are self-satisfied. What we must say, rather, is that they can take the frailties and sins, weaknesses and evils of human nature in the same unquestioning spirit that one takes or accepts the characteristics of nature. (Maslow, 1950)

For Maslow – at least for 'healthy individuals' – self-awareness was as much a process of self-acceptance as anything. It may just be possible that only those who are troubled by their own personalities concentrate very hard on the development of self-awareness. Perhaps the others simply get on with life. This sentiment can be summarized by reference to two other authors. It is summed up by Colin Wilson (1965), who wrote as follows: 'People do not spend their time weighing up existence in order to get through the average working day ...'. It is illustrated, too, by a story in a book by Postman and Weingartner (1971). The story concerns a teacher in a ghetto school in the United States who asked a young child; 'How many legs has a grass-hopper got?' The little boy shook his head rather sadly and replied: 'Gee, man, I wish I had *your* problems ...'. We should, perhaps, make sure that we do not confuse self-awareness and self-indulgence.

Developing self-awareness

With those cautionary comments in mind, it is possible to describe various ways of developing self-awareness. Some involve introspection and some entail involvement with and feedback from other people. Any course leading towards self-awareness must contain both facets: the inner search and the observations of others. Introspection by itself can lead to a one-sided, totally subjective view of the self. It is difficult, if not impossible, for the person working on her own to transcend herself and take the larger view. In order to balance that subjective view, we need the view of others.

Before examining some of the methods of introspection and group work, it is useful to note one simple method of enhancing self-awareness: the process of noticing what we are doing, the process of self-monitoring. All that is involved here is that you stay conscious of what you are doing,

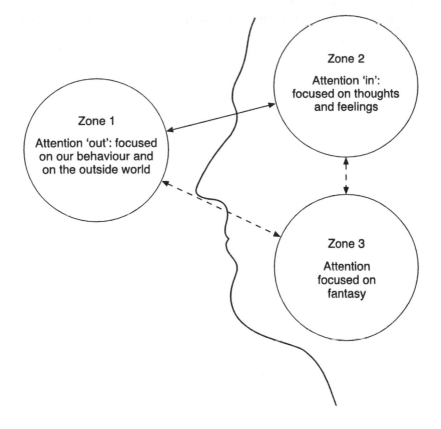

Figure 1.3 Zones of attention

as you do it. In other words, you 'stay awake' and develop the skill of keeping your attention focused on your actions, both verbal and non-verbal. Such a process, whilst easy in theory can, in practice, be quite difficult. It is easy to become distracted by inner thoughts and preoccupations so that our actions become automatic and unnoticed – even robotic. At this point it may be useful to examine three zones of attention on which we can focus.

Figure 1.3 shows these three, hypothetical, zones. Zone 1 is the zone of having our attention focused 'out' – on to our behaviour or on to the world outside of ourselves. This is the zone being described above. To stay awake is to have attention focused outwards. There are some simple devices, borrowed from meditation, that can encourage, enhance or develop our ability to keep our attention in that zone. Here is a straightforward one. Stop reading for a moment and allow your eyes to focus on an object in the room that you are in: it may be a piece of furniture, a picture or anything else that is on hand. Focus your attention on that object and notice every detail of it: its shape, its texture, its colour and so on. Continue to do this for about 30 seconds. Then discontinue your close observation. Notice how, whilst doing the exercise, your attention has been drawn away from your own thoughts and feelings to enable you to focus fully on the object.

The practice of this simple exercise can help in getting and keeping attention 'out'. If we do not focus out, we do not fully notice ourselves and others. Instead, we give half of our attention to ourselves or others and are not really 'present' for either. When we have our attention out, we can give ourselves more fully to what we are doing or give our attention more fully to the person we are with.

Zones 2 and 3 in Figure 1.3 are the zones of introspection. Inward focusing of attention (or 'attention in') can be useful as a means of exploring thoughts, feelings or bodily sensations. Access to Zone 2 is very straightforward. Stop reading and close your eyes. Allow your attention to range freely over what is going on in your mind. Notice the things that you are thinking; notice how you are feeling and pay attention to any body sensations that you have. What parts of your body are you aware of? What parts can you not sense at all? Is there anything you can do in order to become aware of those parts of your body? After one or two minutes, open your eyes and switch your focus back to the outside world. Notice whether such a switch is easy or difficult. The ability to shuttle between Zones 1 and 2 can be developed through practice.

Zone 3 involves fantasy. Fantasy refers to all our thoughts and feelings that involve imagining or day-dreaming: anything that is not *fact*. Notice how we often have fantasies about both ourselves and others that are in no way related to fact. We *imagine* for instance what other people think of us. We *imagine* what sorts of people other people are. We *guess* at what they are thinking about or what they think of us. In each case we are dealing, not with how things *are* but *how we imagine them to be*. Often these imaginings or fantasies are based on the flimsiest of evidence. Often they are pure fantasy – they have no grounding in fact at all! Differentiating between Zones 2 and 3 is particularly fruitful. Such differentiation allows us to distinguish between what we know and what we *think* we know. If we acknowledge when we are moving from the zones of logical, clear thinking (Zone 2) to the zone of fantasy (Zone 3), we develop a clearer picture of what goes on inside our heads. This is not to denigrate the zone of fantasy, for it can be a rich source of creativity and inspiration. It is just to note that fantasy is always just that: it can never be reality.

Awareness of our focus of attention and its shift between the three zones has implications for all aspects of nursing. The nurse who is able to keep her attention focused out for longer periods is likely to become more observant and more accurate in those observations. The nurse who can differentiate between the zones of thinking and the zones of fantasy is less likely to jump to conclusions about her observations or to make value judgements based on prejudice rather than on fact. She is also likely to be more effective as a critical thinker and more able to assess and evaluate new ideas and new theories.

The study of the three zones can never be exhaustive. To explore zone 1 is also to explore the outer aspect of self: our behaviour, speech and so on. It is also to explore the environment in which we live and move. It is to come to know more about the world around us and the people who share it with us.

To explore zone 2 is also a job for life. There would seem to be no end to how much we can study our thought processes, feeling states and bodily sensations. Likewise, examining our fantasy life can give us insights into the sorts of people we are, how we picture ourselves, others and the world around us.

All such explorations can be carried out either in isolation, with another person or in groups. To explore the self in the company of another person can be a rewarding and economical method. Economical in that the time available can be equally divided between the two people. Co-counselling offers a useful format for such exploration and this is explained in the next chapter.

Other methods of self-awareness training include the use of role-play, social skills training, meditation and assertiveness skills training. These methods are well documented in the literature (see for example Kagan, 1985; Bond, 1986; Hargie *et al.*, 1987; Burnard, 1989a) and courses in these forms of training are frequently organized by women's groups, growth centres and extra-mural departments of colleges and universities.

In nurse education and training, the use of video can enhance self-awareness by allowing students to view themselves as if from another person's point of view. Such training, however, should always be voluntary. Some people find the use of video taping a gross invasion of personal territory and the method should be used with discretion.

As we have noted, work on the body via Reichian bodywork, yoga, tai chi, the martial arts and sport all have their place in self-awareness development both for their effects on the body but also for their limit-testing capacity. A quieter, more reflective approach is the use of journals or diaries and these can be used to monitor self-awareness development alongside educational development.

Probably the ideal is a combination of a variety of approaches: introspection, with a group, active and passive. In this way, the self is studied in all its aspects and in a variety of contexts. As we have noted, the 'self' is not a static once-and-for-all thing but an entity that is constantly changing depending, amongst other things, on the people we are with. The eclectic approach is also healthier in that it encourages the combination of sport and exercise alongside meditation and more reflective practices. It also allows for normal social relationships to develop alongside periods of solidarity. No one ever became self-aware by shutting themselves away from the rest of the world. Also, it is important that self-awareness development has a practical end – the enhancement of interpersonal relationships and skills.

Is it really possible to 'know yourself'?

There is a real paradox in trying to get to know yourself better and it is a paradox well known to researchers who try to use themselves as the subject of their own research. It is simply that the person who seeks self-awareness is both seeker and finder. He or she is both doing the looking and the seeing at the same time. The subject of scrutiny is the person who is doing the scrutinizing. All of these ways of putting it point to the same thing: that it is impossible to *detach* yourself *from* yourself to any real degree. To do so would means standing outside of yourself – presumably an impossibility.

On the other hand, this does not mean that *some* self-awareness is not possible but simply that the idea of coming to know yourself *completely* would seem to be out of the question. Clearly, the fact that we receive feedback about ourselves from others means that we can gain some awareness. It could be argued, of course, that such awareness is not *self-*awareness at all but *other* awareness. When another person gives us feedback, he or she does not really tell us about ourselves but tells us *their view of us* – a slightly different point of view. Nevertheless, that information can help us to think about how we see ourselves. We must remain humble about the task that lies ahead of us and not get too satisfied, too quickly, that we have made great strides in the self-awareness process.

Self-awareness and the nurse

Having explored the concept of self and examined some methods of self-awareness development, the question remains: why develop self-awareness anyway?

In the first instance, to discover more about ourselves is to differentiate ourselves from others. If we cannot differentiate between *our own* thoughts and feelings and those of others, we stand to blur our ego boundaries, our sense of our self as an independent, autonomous being. Conversely, if we constantly blur the distinction between 'you and me' we risk not recognizing the other person's independence and autonomy. When ego boundaries are blurred, we lose the sense of whose problem is whose. With self-awareness we can learn to distinguish between our problems and those of others and vice versa. This is particularly important in sensitive areas such as psychiatry and care of the dying person. Real involvement and care in these fields also involves (almost paradoxically) the ability to detach ourselves a little in order to get things into perspective. If we cannot engage in this distancing we risk being drawn into other people's problems to such a degree that we can no longer help them. *Their* problems, have become *ours*.

To become self-aware is also to learn conscious use of the self. We become agents: we are able to choose to act rather than feeling acted upon. We learn to select therapeutic interventions from a range of options so that the patient or client benefits more completely. If we are blind to ourselves we are also blind to our choices. We are blind, then, to caring and therapeutic choices that we could make on behalf of our patients.

Once we can combine two aspects – differentiation from others and an increased awareness of the range of therapeutic choices available to use – we can be more sensitive to the needs and wants of others. We can even choose to *forget ourselves* in order to give ourselves more completely to others. No longer do we run the risk of getting sucked into other people's problems, nor do we confuse *our* thoughts and feelings with those of our patients. We can offer therapeutic distance with therapeutic choice.

Interpersonal interventions such as counselling and group facilitation require that we exercise some self-awareness. All that has been discussed in the above paragraphs is particularly true when we are trying to help people in these particular sorts of therapeutic situations. Later in this book, both counselling skills and group facilitation skills are explored. It is a prerequisite that alongside the development of such skills, the person taking part in the activities in this section of the book will also continue to develop self-awareness. Skills development without self-awareness tends to encourage the development of a stilted and unnatural presentation of self. Without self-awareness, the person appears merely to have a set of skills 'tacked on': those skills are used neither sensitively nor consciously but in a robotic and automatic way.

Problems in self-awareness development

It is worth repeating the point made at various stages throughout this chapter that the aim of self-awareness development is to enable us to increase our interpersonal skills. The path to such awareness is, however, fraught with problems. First is the problem of egocentricity. It is possible to become caught up in the idea of understanding the self to the degree that it becomes an end in itself. This tends to lead to the person becoming self-indulgent and self-centred. Clearly such positions are not compatible with altruism or concern for others. Second, it is possible for those who develop self-awareness to believe that they have discovered insights that set them apart or even make them better than other people. A sign of such development is sometimes the loss of a sense of humour. Life becomes very earnest. True self-awareness, however, tends to lead to a lightness of touch and a sense of humility at the sheer vastness of the task in hand. To continue with that task, it is important that the person maintains (and exercises) a sense of humour in order to keep sight of the 'larger canvas'. Certainly the best run self-awareness groups are those that offer a 'light' atmosphere. If the atmosphere becomes too heavy and earnest, it is likely to put everyone off. It is certainly not conducive to easy and frank self-disclosure.

Linked to this, is the problem of the self-awareness group facilitator becoming something of a 'guru' figure. As people find things out about themselves, they sometimes tend to imagine that the group facilitator has special qualities that enable him or her to allow this to happen. As a result, those people tend to set up the facilitator as some sort of hero figure. Sometimes the facilitator believes in this image too and ends up acting out the role of guru. Again, caution and humility are keywords. Both group members and facilitator should remember that the facilitator is human, like everyone else. Although I make no gender assumptions in my use of words above, it is my experience (and for whatever reason) it is nearly always men who either set themselves up in the guru role or are set up in it by their groups.

Finally comes the issue of voluntariness. Self-awareness cannot be forced upon people. Facilitators of self-awareness groups would do well to exercise what Heron (1977b) calls the voluntary principle. This is a principle invoked at the beginning of any self-awareness training course and repeated at intervals throughout such a course that no one at any time will have pressure exerted on them to take part, and that everyone takes part in any exercise of their own free will. If self-awareness is about developing autonomy and the exercise of choice, it is important that such autonomy and choice begins with deciding whether or not a given exercise suits them at this time. Accepting and respecting other people's frailties, their reserve and their choice not to disclose aspects of themselves until they are ready, are all part of the process of facilitation. Such understanding on the part of the facilitator will do much to increase the confidence of group members and to create an atmosphere conducive to self-understanding.

Beyond self-awareness

It is, I think, possible to move beyond self-awareness and I offer the following diagram to highlight some of the stages that may be moved through to get to that end. The idea of 'no-self' is an important one in the Buddhist religion, where the ultimate objective is to move completely away from 'attachment' to the world, objects in it and even to the notion of self. It is the ultimate stripping of ego and a sense of 'I'. Arguably, we can all become too attached to who we are, what we are, what we want and what we think we should have. In moving beyond self-awareness we can, I believe, potentially move to a state where 'I' no longer looms so large. We are no longer taken up with what is important for us. In a sense, this can lead, perhaps, to true altruism or care for other people. In losing ourselves, we can give more readily to others, for we have no attachment to personal wants, needs or desires.

Stage one	Unaware
Stage two	Self aware
Stage three	Self acceptance
Stage four	Release from self

Stage one, in this model, represents the state in which we do not consider our thoughts, actions and sense of being in any particular way. We are taken up, in an immediate sort of way, with our own wants and needs. We do not reflect particularly closely on our behaviour. In stage two, through various means (some of which are described in this book) we begin to develop a stronger and more secure sense of self. We are more aware of what we are thinking, feeling and doing and more aware of the effect that we have on others. This, in turn, leads to our accepting ourselves for who we are and to our taking responsibility for our actions (although whether we can take full responsibility for our thoughts and feelings remains a moot point). Finally, I think, we can reach a point, in stage four, where – to a greater or lesser degree – we begin to lose an attachment to self. As described above, we no longer find it necessary to ponder on ourselves. Instead, we gradually lose the sense of an individual 'I' and, instead, acknowledge more fully, our oneness with other people. For I suspect that in 'Western', capitalistic societies, we have become overly preoccupied with individuals and their separate wants, needs and desires. This idea is, perhaps, captured well in the Japanese concept of *sabi* – a term that does not easily translate but which is attempted as follows:

> *Sabi* is: a sense of the transitoriness of all things tinged always with sadness; it is felt in solitude; it includes a sense of spontaneity, of all things occurring without relation to others; it is a sense of deep illimitable quietude; it is more readily experienced when we are older, when it comes without being sought; *sabi* has to do with a particular atmosphere, arising from a scene that need not involve a human being, and this atmosphere is generated when something fulfils its destiny in the vast expanse of the universe. To see a creature experiencing its destiny of transience gives rise to *sabi*. *Sabi* is not the English loneliness which suggests a state of inward drabness; rather *sabi* is a state of being alone in which we are not lonely, but are in a state in which we and all things interpenetrate. Hence *sabi* can be said to have to do with the merging of the temporal with the eternal, the mutable with the immutable. *Sabi* involves the belief that one attains perfect spiritual serenity by immersing oneself in the egoless life of nature and it has a connection with the concept of nirvana, the state in which all things are experienced as they really are, empty. (Wilkinson, 2000)

Self-disclosure

The act of telling others important things about ourselves is known as *self-disclosure*. How much we are prepared to share ourselves with others depends on a number of things, including, at least: the degree to which we know the other person, the degree to which we trust them, our affiliation with them, our liking of them and so on. Murray Cox (1978) offered a useful analysis of disclosure when he described three levels of it. First level disclosures include fairly trivial and 'safe' things such as 'I'm fairly hot at the moment' or 'I live on the other side of the town'. Second level disclosures are disclosures of *feelings* and Cox argues that we only make such disclosures once we have got to know and trust the other person a little more. Third level disclosures are those of deep, existential feelings and thoughts. Such disclosures are made only to a few people – if to any at all. If you reflect for a moment on the sorts of things that *you* know about yourself but which you would be hesitant to share with others, you will be able to identify your own third level material. The important thing to bear in mind is that people differ in the *content* of third level disclosures. What may be difficult for me to disclose may be easy for you and vice versa.

Sidney Jourard (1959, 1961, 1964) was one of the pioneers in self-disclosure research. He argued that *self-disclosure begets self-disclosure*. Thus, if I am prepared to share something of myself with you, you are more likely to share part of yourself with me. If Jourard is right, this has interesting implications for nursing and counselling. Both of those relationships, typically and traditionally, depend on one person (the patient or client) self-disclosing to another (the nurse or counsellor) but rarely is there any reciprocation of any depth. Perhaps the balance needs to be redressed and perhaps nurses should consider whether or not they should be prepared to share themselves more with their patients and clients.

The study discussed below was a direct replication of a Jourard study from 1961 in which he used a questionnaire to explore levels of self-disclosure in a small group of university nursing students and the replication was carried out by the author and a colleague, Paul Morrison. We were able to replicate, almost exactly, his 1961 study of 25 British female university students with a mean age of 19.88 and an age range of 18–25 years. All subjects in Jourard's study were unmarried and were classified as middle class. Jourard gave all subjects a 25-item questionnaire which asked respondents about the level of information that they disclosed to four important people in their lives – their mother, their father, a closest male friend and closest female friend.

Jourard found that there was an important tendency for females to disclose more to other females than to males. When comparing his British findings with a comparable sample of American students, Jourard also noted that the American students were generally more disclosing than were the British. Thus the American students had a higher mean disclosure rating than did the British respondents. The American students also had a significant tendency to disclose more to females than to males. In rank order, the students in the British study disclosed most to their mothers, then to their closest female friends, then to their fathers and lastly to their closest male friends. Overall, Jourard also noted a similarity between the American group and the British group in terms of the relative disclosability of certain questionnaire items to certain target persons.

Aims

The aim of the study was to replicate the British element of Jourard's 1961 study. We wanted to know the degree to which a study conducted 30 years after Jourard's would show similarities and differences in terms of self-disclosure amongst young, female university students. We planned to make a direct comparison between our findings and those reported by Jourard.

Sample and data collection

Twenty-five female undergraduate nursing students in a UK university were asked to complete Jourard's 25 item questionnaire. The mean age of the group was 19.72 and the range was 18–23 years. This was an opportunistic sample (Field and Morse, 1985) of 25 students drawn from a larger pool of 32 students because they fell within the age range of the students in Jourard's sample. We asked the group of 25 students to complete the questionnaire that Jourard had used in his 1961 study. In a 1971 publication, Jourard reproduced the questionnaire in full and gave permission for the questionnaire to be used in future studies. The questionnaire was completed by reading 25 statements pertaining to items of personal information and then rating the degree to which the respondent felt that they had disclosed those items of information to their mother, father, same sex and opposite sex friend. Examples of the items of information in the questionnaire included:

- The food you like best and the way that you like the food prepared.
- Whether or not you belong to any church.
- Details of your sex life at the present time.

Very minor modifications to the wording of the questionnaire were made in order to suit the British sample. An example of one such wording change is as follows. Item 10 of Jourard's questionnaire read: 'Whether or not you belong to any clubs, fraternity, civic organizations; if so, the names of these organizations.' We changed this to read: 'Whether or not you belong to any clubs, if so, the names of those clubs.' We anticipated that this would not make a considerable difference to the outcome of the study but that it would aid our respondents' understanding of the questionnaire.

Analysis

Once the 25 respondents had filled in their response sheets we were able to calculate the frequencies of responses to particular items and the number of disclosures to target persons (mother, father, same sex, opposite sex friends). This type of analysis mirrored closely that reported by Jourard and thus allowed us to make a direct comparison with his original findings.

Findings

Two types of score are offered here. These summarize the patterns of disclosure with regard to the target persons and the pattern of disclosures for individual respondents. A little later in the paper we examine the relative disclosability of particular questionnaire items for the group. In Table 1.1 it can be seen that the same sex friend achieved the highest number of disclosures and the father figure received the lowest across the group. The mean scores summarize the overall trend but the range of scores suggests considerable variation within the sample.

The mean scores were also plotted against Jourard's reported figures and a direct comparison could be made. Mean scores of disclosures, across the range of target persons, were higher in the 1991 than in the 1961 study. Also, the ordering of numbers of disclosures to target persons

Table 1.1 Summary of findings from student group in the 1991 study ($n = 25$)

	Target persons			
	Mother	*Father*	*Same sex friend*	*Opposite sex friend*
Total number of disclosures	417	316	447	388
Range	5–22	3–22	10–25	6–25
Mean*	17	13	18	16

*All mean scores have been rounded up.

was different in the two studies. The 1991 group said that they disclosed more frequently to their opposite sex friends than to their fathers. Rank ordering of disclosure levels in the 1991 study was mother, female friend, male friend and father. This can be compared to the rank ordering of disclosure levels in the 1961 study which was mother, female friend, father and male friend.

In addition, the patterns of self-disclosure for individual respondents were identified by examining the total number of disclosures made by each student to all of their significant others (Table 1.2).

A few observations may be made about these patterns of disclosure. First, some respondents appeared to disclose quite highly to all four target persons. For example, respondent 21 had a total score of 78 disclosures. The range of those disclosures was 18–21. The total score suggests that, relative to other respondents, she was a 'high discloser'. The narrow range suggests that she was comfortable disclosing all types of things to all four target persons. On the other hand some respondents appeared to be more selective about who they disclosed to even though they could be regarded as high disclosers in comparison to other respondents. For example, respondent 23 had a total score of 73 disclosures. The range of those disclosures was 14–25. The total score, again, suggest that she was a 'high discloser', but she appeared to be much more selective about which target persons she disclosed to. In this particular instance, the respondent disclosed only 14 items to her father whilst being prepared to disclose all items to her same sex friend.

There are other issues here. Some respondents, for example, were prepared to disclose *all* items to at least one target person, whilst others would not disclose certain items to *any* of the target persons. This highlights some of the subtle issues that are at stake in the study of self-disclosure. It is not simply a matter that some people can be designated 'high disclosers' and others 'low disclosers'. It would seem from this sort of analysis that at least the following possibilities exist:

- That there are people who will disclose much to all significant others.
- That there are people who will disclose much to selected significant others.
- That there are people who will not disclose much to any significant others.

Table 1.2 Pattern of student disclosures ($n = 25$)

Respondent	Total no. of disclosures	Range	Mean
1	62	8–20	15.5
2	70	15–19	17.5
3	53	6–18	13.25
4	48	4–17	12
5	62	6–25	15.5
6	79	18–21	19.75
7	59	7–25	14.75
8	58	8–20	14.5
9	64	13–23	16
10	66	12–19	16.5
11	80	17–24	20
12	57	11–22	14.25
13	74	14–25	18.5
14	57	13–16	14.25
15	53	10–15	13.25
16	72	7–23	18
17	41	5–17	10.25
18	63	12–20	15.75
19	55	3–21	13.75
20	50	9–21	12.5
21	78	18–21	19.5
22	81	17–22	20.25
23	73	14–25	18.25
24	49	4–18	12.25
25	61	12–19	15.25

• That there are people who will disclose a considerable amount to significant others but will not disclose *certain* things.

This analysis raises questions about what determines whether or not a person discloses things about his or herself and what factors affect the likelihood of such disclosure. Also, what influences the *context* of disclosure? How do people make decisions about to whom they will disclose certain issues and not others? All of these questions have significance for both those who work in the 'disclosing professions' such as counselling, nursing and psychotherapy and also have significance for further research into self-disclosure. The issue seems to be a multi-faceted one and requires further study to clarify some of the issues we have outlined here.

These, then, are some of the issues involved in any debate about self and self-awareness. It is necessary to reiterate the fact that this chapter does not include all of the issues that are involved. The idea of 'self' remains a complex and, in many ways, an illusive one. It is easy to talk about the self as if we already knew all about it. It is also easy to assume that psychologists have somehow found out some 'truths' about the self and self-awareness. In fact, we probably know very little about either issue. That should not, however, stop us exploring. For one thing seems certain: nursing is all about selves: the self of the nurse and the selves of his or her patients. However, it is probably also true that is possible to *overstate* the importance of individual selves and this is discussed, above, in the section 'Beyond self-awareness'. In the end, we may not be as important, as individuals, as we care to think we are.

2

Experiential Learning

Nurse education has changed in the past few years. Project 2000 courses have combined 'academic' learning with 'practical learning' to ensure that everyone studying to be a nurse gets an education as well as training. Also, the notion of the *reflective* practitioner has become a central one. Experiential learning has become an important tool for the development of nursing skills (Tomlinson, 1985; Kagan *et al.*, 1986; Miles, 1987). This chapter explores the concept of experiential learning. The aim of this chapter is to explore the concept as it applies to nurse education and particularly as it applies to the development of interpersonal skills. It should be noted, at the outset, that the concept has been used in a wide variety of ways in the literature. Examples of the concepts that various writers have used in the context of experiential learning include, amongst others:

- learning by doing the job
- learning from life experience allowing people credits for their life experience in place of formal qualifications when applying for places at university
- adult education
- humanistic education
- education of feelings as well as thoughts
- progressive and radical educational methods
- education to increase political awareness
- non-formal education
- learning through reflection.

Learning by doing the job

This is simply described as learning by doing. Most of us learned a lot about what our jobs involved simply by working ourselves into the role. The process of learning by doing the job *may* involve formal teaching or it may not. It may also involve some 'sitting by Nellie' – learning the job from another person simply by watching what they do. It could be argued that quite a lot of nursing is learned in this sort of way. Evans comments on the changing ways in which people are learning – both through employment and other means:

> The family, the community and the church contribute relatively little to people's learning. Schools and colleges contribute relatively less than they

did. Learning at work either through the nature of employment, or through in-house courses, has increased markedly. (Evans, 1985)

Learning from life experience

It is a cliché to say that life is a learning experience but there is little doubt that we learn through the process of maturation. One version of experiential learning is the process of learning by being in the world in the first place. The process of growing up, of being educated, of working, of having relationships, all helps us to learn. Boud and Pascoe (1978) identify some of the important characteristics of this sort of experiential learning:

1. The involvement of each individual student in his or her own learning (learning activities need to engage the full attention of a student).
2. The correspondent of the learning activity to the world outside the classroom or educational institution (the emphasis being on the quality of the experience, not its location).
3. Learning control over the learning experience (learners themselves need to have control over the experience in which they are engaged so that they can integrate it with their own mode of operation in the world and can experience the results of their own decisions) (Boud and Pascoe, 1978).

It is important to note that not *all* life experience involves learning. It is quite possible, as someone once noted, either to (a) have 20 years' experience or (b) have 1 year's experience repeated 20 times. Learning from life involves a number of things, including, perhaps, reflection, thinking, change and new experiences from which to learn.

Allowing people credits for their life experience in place of formal qualifications when applying for places at university

This is a particular use of the term 'experiential learning'. Increasingly, university departments and colleges are attempting to widen the access gate to education by paying attention to people's prior life and work experience. The notion of the Accreditation of Prior Experiential Learning (APEL) involves a person drawing up a portfolio of their life experience to date and identifying *what* they have learned and *how* they have learned it. The point of drawing up this portfolio is to offer *evidence* that learning from life has taken place and that *this* person at *this* time has a valid argument for joining a particular course – even though he or she does not have the 'formal' qualifications for joining a course.

Increasingly, nurses are required to have diplomas and degrees as evidence of their competence to practise and/or to teach. Given the nature of the profession, many nurses enter nurse training without the required examination passes to qualify them to enter degree programmes.

The APEL process is often a useful one in that it allows those people access to further and higher education.

Norman Evans (1992), an expert in this particular field, offers a detailed and thorough account of how APEL developed and how it can be used in practice. At the time of writing this fourth edition of this book, it is the case that many nursing courses now offer entry to nursing and health care courses through the APEL system – an indication, perhaps, of the growing appreciation of the value of human, experiential learning as a precursor to more formal learning processes.

Adult education

The term *experiential learning* is sometimes used as a synonym for *adult education*. As we shall see, Malcolm Knowles and others have argued that adult learning differs from the learning processes that take place in childhood and that adult learning *needs* are different from those of children. The adult learning approach is discussed in more detail later in this chapter.

Humanistic education

The effects of the humanistic psychology movement have been pervasive, and sometimes *experiential learning* is used to denote those teaching and learning activities that draw upon the theories of Abraham Maslow, Carl Rogers and others in the humanistic psychology movement. It is worth quoting Rogers at some length here, as the type of experiential learning that is discussed in most detail in this chapter *is* the humanistic approach. Rogers summarized the educational aims of the humanistic approach as being concerned with:

- A climate of trust in the classroom in which curiosity and the natural desire to learn can be nourished and enhanced.
- A participatory mode of decision-making in all aspects of learning in which students, teachers, and administrators each have a part.
- Helping students to prize themselves, to build their confidence and self-esteem.
- Uncovering the excitement in intellectual and emotional discovery, which leads students to become life-long learners.
- Developing in teachers the attitudes that research has shown to be most effective in facilitating learning.
- Helping teachers to grow as persons, finding rich satisfaction in their interaction with learners.
- An awareness that, for all of us, the good life is within, not something that is dependent on outside sources (Rogers, 1983).

However, we should note that in the past 20 years, education has become rather more of a commodity than was the case when Rogers was formulating these ideas. At the beginning of the new century, much more emphasis is placed on teaching and learning as a form of 'business' rather than as a human enterprise focusing on the wants and needs of individual students.

Education of feelings as well as thoughts

Experiential learning is often characterized as addressing not only the *cognitive* side of human beings but their *emotional* needs as well. Traditionally, education has been mostly concerned with rationality, research and thought. Experiential learning is sometimes credited with adjusting the balance between the cognitive and the affective domains. As we shall see throughout this book, the two are difficult to separate when the domain of learning includes the development of interpersonal, human skills. Also, it would be wrong for experiential learning to claim a monopoly on the education of feelings. Presumably many other sorts of teaching and learning methods involve feelings, including lectures, recitations, debates, poetry readings and so on – although none of these, traditionally, would necessarily be thought of as 'experiential learning methods'.

Progressive and radical educational methods

Some versions of experiential learning have argued that it is *progressive* as opposed to *traditional* in its outlook. This particular approach to education owes much to the American educational system and can be traced back to the works of the pragmatic philosopher and educationalist John Dewey. It is worth reflecting on the ways in which all forms of experiential learning differ from traditional, pedagogic frameworks. Cowan and Garry characterize such traditional frameworks like this:

- They do not actively set out to relate that which is learnt to that which is already understood (this is particularly true beyond the specific bounds of the topic being covered).
- No serious attempt is made within the programme to identify or to resolve the *total* relevant needs of learners in that participant group.
- Nothing is or can be done to identify or build on relevant experiential learning.
- All participants are treated similarly; and there is a presumption that their learning is, or should be, of a similar nature.

Motivation is, by implication, extrinsic rather than intrinsic, and hence encourages superficial learning (Cowan and Garry, 1986).

Education to increase political awareness

Sometimes, experiential learning is a label for those teaching activities that help people to become aware of their *political* situation and context. In this case, the aim is to *liberate* and *empower* such people. One of the leading proponents of this approach to learning is Paulo Freire. He notes (Freire,

1974) that, traditionally, there is a teacher–student contradiction that can be characterized as follows:

- The teachers teach but students are taught.
- Teachers are supposed to know everything while students are presumed to know nothing.
- Teachers are supposed to think while students are supposed to be thought about.
- Teachers choose and enforce their choice and students comply in turn.
- Teachers choose the programme contents, and the students, who were not consulted in the first place, adapt to it.
- Teachers become the subject of the learning process while the students become mere objects.

Freire has recommended that learning should become a process of learning through becoming aware of one's social and political situation. To this end, he identifies a *problem-posing* approach to education in which learning takes place through *dialogue* between students and teachers and in which the power imbalance between the two is – at least to some degree – resolved.

It should be noted, however, that much of Freire's writing was concerned with the emancipation and education of workers in South America who had no formal education and who were unaware of the political context in which they were contained. It seems to this writer to be a rather odd thing to attempt to transpose Freire's ideas directly onto the educational canvas of nurse education in the UK, Europe and North America. It has even become popular to talk of nurses being 'oppressed' – in the Freirian sense of the word – and, again, to this writer, this would seem something of a hyperbole. Nurses may have had to fight to gain recognition, in their own right, from the medical profession but this hardly qualifies them to be described as 'oppressed'.

Non-formal education

Beside formal educational courses in colleges and universities, there is a whole host of short, part-time and weekend courses that are not, necessarily, certificated. These include evening courses and weekend workshops and all of these have also been described as *experiential* in nature.

There is another side to non-formal education and that is learning through the process of being involved with the world – however that 'world' is defined. It is the process of learning *outside* of the classroom, college or educational institution. Lindeman (1956) summarizes something of this approach when he writes as follows:

> Learning which is combined with action provides a peculiar and solid enrichment. If, for example, you are interested in art, you will gain much more if you paint as well as look at pictures and read about the history of art. If you happen to be interested in politics, don't be satisfied with being a spectator: participate in political action. If you enjoy nature, refuse to be content with the vicarious

experiences of naturalists: become a naturalist yourself. In all of these ways learning becomes an integral part of living until finally the old distinction between life and education disappears. In short, life itself becomes a perpetual experience of learning. (Lindeman, 1956)

Lindeman is claimed by a number of writers (Jarvis and Knowles amongst them) to be one of the seminal writers on adult education and a educationalist whose work anticipated the experiential learning movement.

Learning through reflection

We can go through life *noticing* what happens to us or we can go through life on 'automatic pilot' – simply *doing* things. Arguably, if we want to *change* our behaviour we have, first, to notice what we do and then *reflect* on our reasons for doing it. The ability to reflect is an essential part of becoming an expert practitioner in nursing. This idea of reflection is so central that the whole of the next chapter is dedicated to it.

The one thing that all of these various ways of approaching experiential learning have in common is the centrality of human experience as a valued source of learning. What follows is an attempt to explore ways in which we might learn from that experience. It is notable, too, that many of the writers who define experiential learning in so many different ways tend to refer to the work of David Kolb (1984), whose experiential learning cycle will be examined in this chapter.

Learning by experience

We all learn through experience, whether directly through taking action, through being involved in a situation or by observing others. In this sense, every situation is a potential learning situation. If we are not careful, the definition could become life = experiential learning and the definition would be so broad as to be of little meaning. It may be more helpful if we can pin it down a little more.

The first thing to note is that whilst every situation is a *potential* learning situation, we do not necessarily learn from everything we do or everything that we are involved in. Some sort of *cognitive* process is required: we need to notice what we do and we need to be aware of what is happening; thus, the emphasis on self-awareness in the previous chapter. To learn more about ourselves (and then to learn about others), a basic requirement is that we *notice* ourselves. We need to be both *reflective* and able to notice what is happening around us and also *reflexive*, able to look inward and notice what we are thinking and feeling. Figure 2.1 offers a simple model of experiential learning which brings together these two notions of experience followed by reflection and adds another ingredient: the transformation of knowledge.

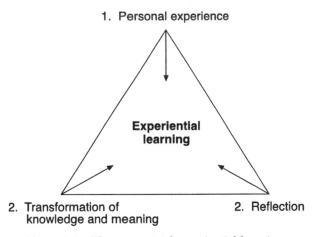

Figure 2.1 The concept of experiential learning

First, the concept involves personal experience – the fact that something has happened to us, or our being actively involved in a situation. Such experience involves the whole of us: our thinking, feeling, behaving and bodily sense. The concept of personal experience can be loosely defined as our involvement in a situation.

The second element of experiential learning is the process of reflection. Often as something happens to us, we may have reason to ponder on it. We may not. Things may happen to us that we either do not notice or we quickly dismiss. Think for a moment of the times that you have driven (or been driven) from one place to another and then wondered how you had got from A to B. You did not realize what was happening because you did not *notice*: you were on 'automatic driver'. In experiential learning, the reflective process is vital. It is only through such refection that we can ever achieve the third element: the transformation or knowledge and meaning.

Experiential learning can be characterized in at least two ways: (a) as an attitude towards learning and (b) as an approach to the question 'What is knowledge?' These two issues are now discussed.

An attitude towards learning

Many traditional methods of teaching and learning offer students large chunks of pre-packaged knowledge in indigestible chunks, upon which no reflection can take place. It is as if the object of learning was to be filled with knowledge, which can, at a later date, be cashed out through examinations. Paulo Freire, the radical Marxist educator (Freire, 1970, 1972) has referred to this as the 'banking' concept of knowledge. Knowledge is fed into the person, who reproduces it, later, in a relatively unchanged state. The main aim is to satisfy your educators that you have absorbed enough. Such an approach, apart from being fairly dull and unimaginative, presupposes a particular view of the nature of knowledge. From this traditional, 'banking' approach, aspects of knowledge are unchanging: 'facts are facts' and they exist independently of the one who does the 'knowing'. The process of education, then, is the initiation of the person into 'ways of knowing' (Peters, 1972). Educators are the 'ones who know' and students are the ones who don't. The educated person, presumably, is the one who has absorbed more knowledge than the rest.

An alternative approach is that which constantly questions knowledge. One of Marx's favourite aphorisms was 'doubt everything' (Singer, 1980) and this characterizes what Paulo Freire calls the 'problem-posing' approach to education (Freire, 1972). Rather than accepting everything that is passed on through traditional methods of teaching and learning, this approach emphasizes an approach to constantly questioning what is learnt through reference to *one's own* experience of the world. In other words, the 'received' view of the world is constantly called into question. Much of traditional nurse education has favoured the unquestioning acceptance of things as they are. The problem-posing approach calls for challenge, doubt and an ability to question the established order to things. This ability to question the traditional and the accepted is demonstrated by two statements that Carl Rogers makes (Rogers, 1967): 'I can trust my experience' and 'evaluation by others is not a guide for me'. Here, the accent is on finding out for one's self: of testing out established theory through one's own experience.

How, then, can nurse educators encourage the development of critical ability? Drawing from and developing the work of Brookfield (1987), the following guidelines are offered.

1   Affirm critical thinkers' self worth

Critical thinkers are innovators. They go out on a limb trying to question the established order of things. They also challenge their own self-concept. For what we think and feel, as we have noted, constitutes our sense of self. We are our knowledge, feelings and actions. For these reasons, critical thinkers need to be encouraged and made to feel that their ideas are appreciated and valued. In the exercises that follow, it is important that unusual ideas are also listened to.

2   Listen attentively to critical thinkers

Listening is an important aspect of nursing practice. We will see in the next chapter that it is one of the most important skills in counselling. It is also a prerequisite for helping to develop critical ability. Someone who is expressing critical ideas is challenging the status quo and offering new views on a particular situation. The temptation is to react – to attempt to bring the student back to the well-worn path. The facilitator who listens, however, develops the ability to follow a critical student's thought processes and enters that person's 'frame of reference' (Rogers, 1967). Such listening is always a challenge, for what we may hear, when we listen to critical expression, may challenge our own view of the world. This notion of an expanding frame of reference is at some variance with traditional views of education. Peters (1972), for example, argues that education is 'initiation into ways of knowing' and that the teacher's task is to lead the student into fields of study. In the version offered here, both students and teachers are co-travellers and develop their knowledge, feelings and skills alongside each other. Each challenges the other.

3 Be a critical teacher

A number of writers on education have discussed the notion of critical teaching. Shor (1980) defines critical teaching as assisting people to become aware of their taken-for-granted world. In the problem-posing and critical approach to experiential learning, the facilitator acts as a catalyst, challenging students to develop their new ideas and to question the world they find themselves in. Freire (1986) has suggested that the characteristics of such facilitators include: competence, courage, risk-taking, humility and political clarity.

Setting out to engage in an experiential learning session of this sort is something of an act of faith. There is no way of knowing beforehand how such a session will end. Either students or facilitator, or both, may change their ideas as a result of the session. The facilitator who practises in this way 'lives on the edge' and is prepared to take risks both with herself and with her students, in order to move thinking and feeling forward. The other important point here is that 'critical facilitation' does not involve the facilitator being critical of the student, as might be the case in more traditional teaching. Indeed, the notion represents almost the opposite position. The facilitator is accepting of the student but prepared to question both her own and the student's ideas.

4 Model critical ability

If students are to learn to question and to criticize, it is important that facilitators demonstrate their own critical ability. This requires that the facilitator stays open to new ideas herself and continues her own educational practice. In this sense, the facilitator, too, stays open to learning from the students. Thus nurse education can become a reciprocal process: students and teachers switch roles throughout the educational process – a notion that Freire has also frequently referred to in his writings (Freire, 1970, 1972, 1985).

5 Learn to shut up!

Most nurse teachers talk too much. If facilitators are to encourage critical ability, students must have the chance to talk about what they think and feel. This cannot happen if the facilitator is talking. Further, silence has much to commend it. The notion that the facilitator must always 'fill in the gaps' during an educational encounter may be an erroneous one.

6 Be conversational

Much can be achieved if the facilitator adopts a fairly normal tone of voice and relates to students as equals and as interesting people with ideas of their own. Many interviews are spoiled by the artificial manner adopted by interviewers (Zweig, 1965). Many potential learning encounters are also spoiled by the teacher too zealously playing out a 'teacher role'. Much of the learning we do takes place outside of educational institutions (Illich, 1973) and this may be because in everyday life, people talk to each other normally. A conversational exchange in the classroom can do much to enhance the free development of critical awareness in students. This notion of 'speaking normally' is an important one in experiential learning. In a field that has attracted a number of 'guru' figures, it is important that experiential learning facilitators take care not to mystify or otherwise worry their students.

This idea of being conversational can also apply to the written word. In the past few years, nursing *literature* has become increasingly obscure in its use of language and this is often to the detriment of understanding. Just as it is important to use simple and clear language when we *speak*, so it is vital that we use such language when we *write*. Writing – of all sorts – is a form of communication. If we really want to convey ideas to other people we need to use language that is accessible.

7 Be normal

Teachers do not have to occupy superior positions to their students. Just because you happen to occupy the role of 'teacher' does not, automatically, make you a cleverer or more competent person than those whom you teach. While there are all sorts of cultural and power factors at work in the relationship between teachers and students it seems to be important that teachers remain 'ordinary' and accessible. Once we, as teachers, believe that we 'know' something special to which students do not have access, we do, I think lose a certain humanity.

On the other hand, we should not underestimate the difficulties attached to stepping down from the teacher role. It is one thing for a teacher to acknowledge to his students that 'Look! I am just like you!' and quite another for students to accept and acknowledge that fact. We should not deny the strength of the socialization process which leads students to believe that teachers occupy a different position to the one they occupy themselves. Nor, perhaps, should we lose sight of the fact that there is usually an age difference between teachers and their students. Teachers should not be in a rush to dismiss that difference. It is probably true that while teachers would often like to be seen as 'colleagues' to their students, those students may be in no particular hurry to welcome teachers to that role. Teachers, can, however, do much to indicate that they are 'normal' and 'ordinary' to their students and it is to be hoped that this, in turn, will lead to a great equality between the roles of nurses and health care professionals and their patients. For, in the past, medics and nurses tended to keep themselves at a distance from their patients – just as teachers distanced themselves from their students. Such power-play led to doctors being viewed as 'gods' and nurses as 'angels'. In bridging this distance between health care professionals and their patients we can do much, I think, to help patients acknowledge their own responsibility in the personal health care arena and lessen dependence on health care professionals as 'those in the know'.

Experiential learning as the development of experiential knowledge

Another approach to appreciating the notion of experiential learning comes through the notion of types of knowledge. Three types of knowledge that go to make up an individual may be described: propositional knowledge, practical knowledge and experiential knowledge (Heron, 1981). Whilst each of these types is different, each is interrelated with the other. Thus, whilst propositional knowledge is qualitatively different to, say, practical knowledge, it is possible and probably better to use propositional knowledge in the application of practical knowledge.

Propositional knowledge

Propositional knowledge is that which may be contained in theories or models. It may be described as 'textbook' knowledge and is synonymous with Ryle's (1949) concept of 'knowing that', which is a concept further developed in an educational context by Pring (1976). A person may build up a considerable bank of facts, theories or ideas about a subject, person or thing, without necessarily having any direct experience of that subject, person or thing. A person may, for example, develop a considerable propositional knowledge about, say, midwifery, without ever necessarily having been anywhere near a woman who is having a baby! Presumably it would be more useful to combine that knowledge with some practical experience, but this does not necessarily have to be the case. This, then, is the domain of propositional knowledge. Obviously it is possible to have propositional knowledge about a great number of subject areas ranging from science to literature or from counselling to physiology. Any information contained in books must necessarily be of the propositional sort.

Practical knowledge

Practical knowledge is knowledge developed through the acquisition of skills. Thus changing a dressing or driving a motor bike demonstrates practical knowledge, though, equally, so does the use of counselling skills, which involve the use of specific verbal and non-verbal behaviours and intentional use of counselling interventions as described above. Practical knowledge is synonymous with Ryle's (1949) concept of 'knowing how', which was developed in an educational context by Pring (1976). Usually more than mere 'knack', practical knowledge is the substance of a smooth performance of a practical or interpersonal skill. A considerable amount of a nurse's time is taken up with the demonstration of practical knowledge – often, but not always, of the interpersonal sort.

Most educational programmes in schools and colleges have concerned themselves primarily with both propositional and practical knowledge and particularly the former. Thus the 'propositional knowledge' aspect of a person is the aspect that is often held in highest regard. Practical knowledge, although respected, is usually seen as slightly less important than the propositional sort. In this way, the 'self' can become highly developed in one sense – the propositional knowledge aspect – at the expense of being skilled in a practical sense.

Experiential knowledge

Experiential knowledge is knowledge gained through direct encounter with a subject, person or thing. It is the subjective and affective nature of that encounter that contributes to this sort of knowledge. Experiential knowledge is knowledge through relationship. Such knowledge is synonymous with Rogers' (1983) description of experiential learning and with Polanyi's concept of 'personal' knowledge and 'tacit' knowledge (Polanyi, 1958). If we reflect for a moment we may realize that most of the things that are really important to us belong in this domain. If we consider our personal relationships with other people, we discover that what we like or love about them cannot be reduced to a series of propositional statements and yet the feelings we have for them are vital and part of what is most important in our lives. Most encounters with others contain the possible seeds of experiential knowledge. It is only when we are so detached from other people that we treat them as objects that no experiential learning can occur.

Not that all experiential knowledge is tied exclusively to relationships with other people. For example, I had propositional knowledge about America before I went there. When I went there, all that propositional knowledge was changed considerably. What I had known was changed by my direct experience of the country. I had developed experiential knowledge of the place. Experiential knowledge is not of the same type or order as propositional or practical knowledge. It is, nevertheless, important knowledge, in that it affects everything else we think about or do.

Experiential knowledge is necessarily personal and idiosyncratic. Indeed, as Rogers (1983) points out, it may be difficult to convey to another person in words. Words tend to be loaded with personal (often experiential) meanings and thus to understand each other we need to understand the nature of the way in which the people with whom we converse use words. It is arguable, however, that such experiential knowledge is sometimes conveyed to others through gesture, eye contact, tone of voice, inflection and all the other non-verbal and paralinguistic aspects of communication (Argyle, 1975). Indeed, it may be experiential knowledge that is passed on when two people (for example a nurse and a patient) become very involved with each other in a conversation, a learning encounter or counselling.

From the above discussion of three types of knowledge, it is possible to define experiential learning, another way, as *any learning activity that*

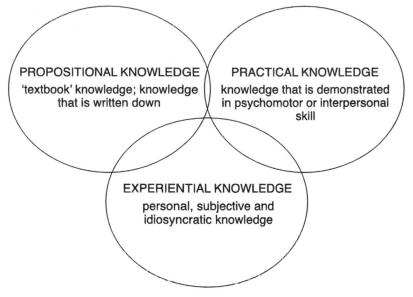

Figure 2.2 Types of knowledge

enhances the development of experiential knowledge. As all interpersonal relationships with others, both within and without the health care professions involve an investment of self, it seems reasonable to argue that any learning methods that involve the self and that involve personal knowledge are likely to enhance personal effectiveness. We cannot, after all, learn interpersonal skills by rote, nor merely by mechanically learning a series of behaviours. We need to spend time reflecting on ourselves and on receiving feedback on our performance from other people.

Figure 2.2 illustrates the interplay between the three types of knowledge described in this section. As we have noted, propositional, practical and experiential forms of knowledge do not exist independently of each other. Each needs to other to 'support' it. Also, in relation to Figure 2.2, we may note that, at different times, an individual might use different types of knowledge in different proportions. Thus the person who is undertaking a degree course might find him or herself more caught up in the 'propositional' domain, whilst the practising clinician may access the 'practical' knowledge domain more frequently. What binds both together, though, is the 'experiential' domain – the domain that 'personalizes' all other types of knowledge.

Learning through and learning from experience

Yet another way of understanding the concept of experiential learning is by the division of *learning through* experience and *learning from* experience. In learning through experience, a situation is set up that allows us to gain insight through participation. In learning *from* experience, we are required to look back at a past situation in our lives in order to glean new meanings from it and to compare it to our present situation. Both types of experiential situation may help us to think critically and carefully about ourselves, our nursing practice and about the *theories* that other people offer us.

The characteristics of experiential learning

It is useful to identify the characteristics that consistently emerge from the theory and practice of experiential learning. These are as follows:

- There is an emphasis on action.
- Students are encouraged to reflect on their experience.
- A clarifying approach is adopted by the facilitator.
- There is an accent on personal experience.
- Human experience is valued as a source of learning.

These characteristics are now examined in order to make further sense of the concept of experiential learning. We have already noted the diversity of the definitions of experiential learning in the literature but these characteristics seem to permeate most approaches to the topic.

There is an emphasis on action

Most experiential learning methods involve the participants in some form of action. This is not to say that they are 'doing something' in a trivial sense but that they are learning through the processes of activity and movement. This can be viewed as the opposite of traditional teaching/ learning strategies which require the learner to be the passive recipient of received knowledge. Through activity we are engaged in learning through all of our senses, not merely in some sort of thinking process. In another sense, too, experiential learning should *lead* to action. If our behaviour does not change as a result of our learning (particularly in the domain of interpersonal skills) then it is arguable that the learning has not been particularly valuable. Also, as we become more critically aware, we will tend to question more and thus want to change what we find in the clinical and community settings.

Students are encouraged to reflect on their experience

Most writers in the field acknowledge that experience alone is not sufficient to ensure that learning takes place. Importance is placed on the integration of new experience with old through the process of reflection (Freire, 1972; Kilty, 1982; Kolb, 1984). In order to learn at all, we must be able to reflect on what we do and to undertake some sort of critical appraisal of what we find. The word 'critical' here is used to denote the process by which we ponder, sift, analyse and evaluate: it should not be taken as meaning only 'to judge negatively'.

Reflection can be a solitary, introspective act or it can be a group process whereby sense is made of an experience through group discussion. If reflection as a group activity is to be successful, the teacher is required to act as a group facilitator. The skills associated with group facilitation differ from those associated with the usual process of teaching in that the group facilitator takes a non-directive and non-authoritarian stance in relation to the students. In a reflective group, the teacher neither ascribes meanings to experience nor offers explanations but allows and encourages the students to do these things for themselves. The issue of reflection in experiential learning is so central that another chapter in this book concentrates *only* on the processes of reflection.

A clarifying approach is adopted by the teacher

In the experiential approach, the teacher does not 'teach' in the traditional sense: he or she does not dispense knowledge or force *their* meanings onto the student's experience (Gray, 1986). Instead, the teacher helps the students to make sense of their *own* experience. After an exercise in which students practise counselling skills, the facilitator encourages quiet reflection on the exercise. Rather than offering explanations for what the students have undergone, the facilitator invites each student to comment on what happened and invites individuals and the group to 'make sense' of what happened. The facilitator may help the students to verbalize their feelings and ideas but he does not attempt to direct them. He may, however, want to challenge them to consider *other* ways of construing what they have experienced. This challenging is an approach to encouraging the students to think in alternative and different ways (Brookfield, 1987). It is vital to critical development. This is not to suggest that the facilitator says 'But there is another way to see this ... here is another theory ...'. Instead, the facilitator merely asks something like 'Are there other ways of looking at this ...? and waits for the students to bring forward other perspectives.

All this is not easy! Teachers, perhaps by nature, like telling students about their own particular experiences or theories. Probably most teachers talk too much. To stand back and allow personal discovery and personal theory development in this way is often to go against the traditional role of the teacher.

Through this process of clarification and critical development, nurses may develop an ability to trust their own judgement and to accept the validity of their own ideas, whilst respecting and appreciating other points of view. They do not strive towards *the* point of view. Nor do they have to defer to the better judgement or knowledge of the teacher but appreciate the value of their own thoughts and feelings about their experiences, both in the school or college and in clinical settings. In this sense, the nurse educator acts as a true 'facilitator of learning'. In the literature on experiential learning, the term 'facilitator' is often used in preference to the terms teacher, tutor and lecturer.

There is an accent on personal experience

Alfred North Whitehead discussed the problem of 'dead' knowledge and asserted that 'knowledge keeps no better than fish!' (Whitehead, 1932). Someone else has described formal teaching as 'dragging a set of old bones from one graveyard to another'. Experiential learning emphasizes the evolving, dynamic, nature of knowledge. Rather than viewing knowledge as fixed and immutable, it stresses the importance of the student understanding and creating a view of the world in that student's own terms. Knowledge, then, is not something that is 'tacked on' to the person: it becomes part of the person themselves. What we learn changes our world-view and changes us. We are what we know. This is what is meant by the accent on personal experience.

As nurses continue through education and training, what they learn becomes part of them. The nurse who becomes skilled at discussing problems with clients or patient changes as a result: the very personal experience of developing human skills helps the nurse towards an enhanced self-concept.

The development of experiential learning methods

Experiential learning methods have evolved from two main sources. One is from the theorizing of the American pragmatic philosopher John Dewey. Dewey argues that all educational processes should be based on the life experiences of the students and that school experiences and life experiences should be directly linked in a planned programme. Dewey was founder of the 'progressive' school of educational thought as opposed of the 'traditional' school which stressed the importance of academic disciples and the impartiality of knowledge. In stressing the importance of life experience as the foundation for the learning process, Dewey anticipated the work of Carl Rogers, Malcolm Knowles and other writers who democratized and personalized learning theory. His emphasis on practicality, the value of experience and the use of the student's own theorizing, made him a key figure in the history of experiential learning theory (Dewey, 1958, 1966, 1971).

The second source from which many experiential learning methods are derived is the school of humanistic psychology. Humanistic psychology developed as a 'third force' in psychology in the 1950s and 1960s. The other two forces were behaviourism and psychoanalysis. Humanistic psychology opposed behaviourism on the grounds that it took a mechanistic view of the human being (although some have argued that the two approaches may be compatible – Woolfolk and Sass, 1989). Psychodynamic psychology was viewed as being overly deterministic. (A deterministic theory is one that argues that present events are necessarily caused by previous events. Thus, for the psychoanalyst, we are a product of our past.) Humanistic psychology opposed this determinism, arguing the idea that people were able to exercise free will and to some degree *choose* who they were. In other words, the person was an 'agent':

not 'acted upon' by her past but freely able to make decisions about herself based on choice.

Thus behaviourism saw people as highly complex machines who could be 'programmed' or subject to positive and negative reinforcement. Psychoanalytic theory saw people as controlled by, and acting out of, their past. Humanistic theory, drawing from existential philosophy, saw people as free decision-makers who could, and usually did, change according to their own wishes.

It can be argued that there are at least two types of humanistic psychology (Mahrer, 1989; Rowan, 1989b). One is the sort that has a particularly positive view of human beings. People, in this approach, are viewed as having a tendency to 'grow' and develop. At its most extreme, this approach argues that people are essentially 'good': an idea that dates back at least to Rousseau. It is an idea that has tended to be a reaction against the Protestant and Freudian notion of people as essentially 'evil' or bad. This 'positive' view of humanistic psychology is typified by writers such as Carl Rogers (1952, 1967) and Abraham Maslow (1972). Maslow, incidentally, is usually credited as being the person who named humanistic psychology.

The second type of humanistic psychology draws more particularly from existentialism and sees people as neither good nor bad. In this version people are completely free. That freedom does not necessarily lead them towards goodness or badness. Essentially, then, people are 'neutral'. Representative writers of this approach include Rollo May (1989) and Erich Fromm (1975, 1979).

Humanistic psychology has as its central focus, the person. Both types acknowledge that people are complex, individual and ever-changing. Thus no *one* theory of how people 'work' would necessarily explain *this* person in *this* situation. Humanistic psychology makes allowance for this variety of human experience. It places great importance on how the individuals interpret their world and does not seek to develop a 'grand theory' of how human beings think, feel and act. This is at some variance with behaviourism and psychoanalysis, both of which offer overall explanatory theories of the person.

This theme of individual, subjective interpretation or experience underpins the thinking behind the exercises in Chapters 6 and 7 of this book. Those exercises do not tell individuals what to expect or what they *should* experience: the emphasis is on the people involved discussing what happened to them as individuals with wide varieties of thoughts, feelings, beliefs and attitudes. After all, we all come to such exercises from different backgrounds. None of our personal histories are the same.

The literature on humanistic psychology is vast (see, for examples, Maslow, 1972; Shafer, 1978; Rowan, 1988, 1989b; Wilber, 1989) and the pros and cons of this approach to psychology will not be discussed here. Suffice to say that humanistic psychology has greatly influenced both nursing and education. Carl Rogers' client-centred counselling (Burnard, 1989c; Rogers, 1967, 1983) has revolutionized the approach to nurse–patient relationships in psychiatric hospitals. This approach gave back to the patients their autonomy and self-direction. It was no longer nurses who made all the decisions but the patients themselves. The humanistic theme has emerged in the revised syllabi of training for general, psychiatric and mental handicap nursing.

The nursing process and nursing models also offer evidence of the impact of humanistic psychology on nursing. These models place the patient at the centre of the nursing profession and emphasize the need for individualized care planning. On the other hand, it should also be noted that many of the nursing theories and nursing models developed between the 1970s and 1990s were not generated from a research base. One of the strengths of nursing as an academic enterprise in the past few years, in my view, has been the appropriate emphasis on nursing having a sound *evidence base*. We must, I think, rely much more on evidence from the research and far less on rather obscure and highly theoretical nursing theories. In the end, we must continue to ask the questions: 'What works in nursing?' and 'What works *best*?' Nor is this a call for any *particular* styles of research. We can use the evidence from both qualitative and quantitative studies to answer these questions. And we should note that the answers to the questions are always going to be changing in the light of new evidence. It is in this cyclical manner of asking questions, finding the answers and posing new questions that we will continue to keep nursing knowledge alive and vibrant. And, in the process, continually enhancing patient care.

Problems with the humanistic approach

Any approach to understanding the person has its problems. Humanistic psychology is no exception. First, humanistic psychology is sometimes argued to be *too* individualistic. Clearly, if everyone's experience was *completely* different to every other person's experience, communication would be impossible! It is important, therefore, to acknowledge the similarities in human experience as well as the differences. A passage attributed to the psychologist Gordon Allport sums up useful positions on this issue:

All persons are, in some ways:

(a) like *all* other people,
(b) like *some* other people,
(c) like other people.

Second, the 'positive' position adopted by some humanistic psychologists has sometimes been attacked as an overly optimistic one. Certainly it can be seen as a direct reaction to other, more negative, positions. As we have noted, there is an alternative position of 'neutrality'. In this position, persons are neither good nor bad: they are free to choose a whole range of behaviours. It is also arguable that 'goodness' and 'badness' are not absolutes but are social constructs. In other words, at different times in history, society dictates what passes as good or bad.

Third, humanistic psychology is sometimes viewed as having had little impact in academic circles. Carl Rogers noted in 1983 that it had never become a real force in psychology courses in universities. Possible reasons for this are various. First, it does not follow the 'scientific' traditions of behavioural psychology (and behavioural psychology has always led the way in psychology departments in most UK universities). Second, because it concentrates so much on *personal* experience and not on generalizations, it is very difficult to identify particular concepts, theories and general propositions about the human situation. This makes for difficulty in establishing a formal 'knowledge base' within the field. Third, and again because of the focus on the individual, traditional, quantitative research methods have not been appropriate for researching the field. Qualitative methods that suit the purpose have only recently emerged and are taking time to establish themselves as valid ones (Reason and Rowan, 1981).

In the next section, a number of humanistic themes and approaches are examined – for two reasons. First, the examination of these themes helps in the understanding of the concepts of both self-awareness and experiential learning. Second, the themes under discussion are often the original sources of the exercises offered later in this book. Once again, the recurring themes will be the importance of individual interpretation of experience, the process of reflection and the value of discussion and of sharing experience.

Examples of humanistic influences in experiential learning

Co-counselling

Co-counselling is a two-way process in which two people take turns to spend time as 'counsellor' and 'client', The client takes time to verbalize and talk through issues and problems from everyday life, while the counsellor gives the client her attention. The counsellor in this relationship does not act in the traditional counselling manner. In other words, she does not offer advice nor attempt to 'sort out' the client. In this self-directed approach the client himself learns to examine his own problems and to 'counsel himself'. Each individual normally spends about 1 hour in the role of counsellor and 1 hour in the role of client. In this way, true interdependence is established. Neither part is wholly dependent upon the other. Responsibility is shared, tough responsibility for working through problems remains firmly with the client. The counsellor may be invited to make interventions at the request of the client, according to a pre-determined contract established between them.

Co-counselling can be used in a variety of ways. It can be a means of de-stressing for nurses working in areas of high emotional involvement. The process of verbalizing pent-up feelings to another person in an understanding and confidential atmosphere can be very therapeutic. Co-counselling can also be used as a means of developing self-awareness through the process of exploring inner thoughts and feelings and particularly buried emotion. It can also be used as a means of practical problem-solving, of talking out personal problems and making decisions about any aspects of the person's life.

Co-counselling developed in the USA under the influence of Harvey Jackins (Jackins, 1965, 1970) and, in this country, John Heron (Heron, 1974, 1978; Heron and Reason, 1981, 1982). It has made its mark within the field of experiential learning. David Potts (in Boud, 1981) has described its use as a learning tool in a university course and James Kilty (1982) has suggested the use of co-counselling in student nurse training. It can be of particular value as a self and peer support system for nurses working in clinical environments that are particularly stressful: intensive care units, children's wards, oncology departments, hospices, psychiatric units and so forth.

Co-counselling training usually takes place through a 40-hour training course, during the course of 1 week, over 2 weekends or through a series of evening classes. Advanced co-counselling and co-counselling teacher training courses are also organized in colleges and extra-mural departments of universities.

Figure 2.3 is a simplified map of the theory behind co-counselling. This is necessarily a simple guide to the theory and the reader is directed to the recommended reading list at the end of the chapter for a more thorough explanation of what is involved.

The assumptions behind co-counselling are that people are potentially autonomous and able to exercise choice. Through the process of living, the individual experiences various types of stress which cause the blocking or repression of emotions. If those blocked emotions can be freed, then the person can once again be capable of making life-decisions and exercising freedom of choice. Co-counselling aims at enabling the individual to express that blocked feeling and thus become more able to be in charge of his or her life.

There are implications, here, for nursing practice. As a general rule, we usually want to calm down people who are frightened, reassure those who are crying and stop people from expressing anger. Could we as nurses be trained to *enable* people to express those emotions as a therapeutic human act? In the fields of psychiatric and mental handicap nursing the value of such an approach is perhaps clear: expressed emotion is presumably better than repressed emotion. It is also of value in general nursing. Pre- and postoperative situations, before and after childbirth, following bereavement, all these situations involve emotional experiences. Nurses can be trained to help their patients to express those feelings freely rather than (a) prematurely stopping them or (b) feeling inadequate and unable to cope. Co-counselling offers one approach to coping with emotion. First, it enables the individual to experience their own emotional feelings and, second, it trains people in handling other people's emotional release.

Co-counselling is a clear example of experiential learning in that it asks the individual to review past and present experience and to reconstruct

1. People are potentially autonomous, self-directing, positive and able to exercise freedom of choice.

↓

2. *However,* people are subject to a variety of stresses throughout life; early childhood experiences, partings, bereavement, difficulties in relationships, spiritual doubts and so forth.

↓

3. Such stresses cause emotions (e.g. fear, anger, grief, embarrassment) to become 'bottled up'.

↓

4. Through talking out and through emotional release (trembling, angry sounds, crying, laughter), those pent-up emotions may be released.

↓

5. Such release generates insight and enables people to think more clearly, to become less rigid, more autonomous and more able to take charge of their lives. They feel less 'acted upon' and more able to exercise choice. They can be spontaneously, positive and life asserting.

↓

6. Co-counselling training, through working in pairs, offers people training in:
   (a) listening to and giving attention to others
   (b) reviewing and re-evaluating life experiences to date
   (c) the release of pent-up emotion (catharsis)
   (d) handling other people's catharsis
   (e) problem-solving and life-planning skills

Figure 2.3   A simple map of the theory of co-counselling

their understanding in the light of the discoveries made. The co-counsel-ling format is simple and can readily be adapted to a variety of learning situations in nurse education. A number of the exercises in given in this book have been developed out of co-counselling training. Liss sum-marizes some of the advantages of the co-counselling approach like this:

> One of the reasons co-counselling works is that it sets the stage of uninter-rupted attention given to one person. Uninterrupted attention is an essential human need and helps the working out of any problem. One of the reasons spouses and friends so often fail to help one another is that they are inclined to interrupt. Not just an interrupting remark, although this itself can break the delicate thread of a talker's stream of consciousness and feeling, but just to interrupt the talker's point of attention can botch up the job. An uncalled for interpretation or unasked for advice will often do this. Even worse is 'This happened to me too ...'. (Liss, 1974)

Liss's summary also makes clear the value of co-counselling in helping a person to develop basic (and perhaps not-so-basic) counselling skills.

The ability to listen, fully, to another person is often described as the basic prerequisite of effective counselling and there are few better ways to learn to listen than through co-counselling.

The co-counselling format can be modified in various ways. The simple pairs method can be used as an introductory activity at the start of a learning session. The group is divided into pairs and one person in each pair talks to the other about whatever is at the forefront of her mind. Her partner listens but does not comment. After 5 minutes, roles are reversed and the 'listener' becomes the 'talker' and vice versa. The pairs format can also be used to explore *particular* issues, e.g. the validity of nursing models to nursing practice or the role of interpersonal skills training in nurse education – any topic that is relevant to the subject under discussion. The format offers an economical and simple method of identifying a wide range of views, thoughts, attitudes and beliefs. It also honours the *student's* views and is not heavily teacher-centred, as are more traditional methods of teaching and learning.

Role play

The use of role play is fairly widespread in nurse education. It relates directly to psychodrama. Psychodrama was devised by the Viennese psychiatrist Jacob Moreno, who advocated the use of dramatic representations of painful, interpersonal events, played out on a stage (Moreno, 1959, 1969, 1977). His new method of therapy enabled people to try out new ways of behaving, to say things that needed saying in real life but which, in real life, were not said. In this way the person was able to rehearse new approaches to life, to try things out and to experiment. Moreno was careful to make the psychodrama realistic and even went so far as to design and build a theatre in which the psychodrama took place. In fact Moreno was the 'inventor' of many of the activities and exercises that later became widely used in self-awareness and therapy groups (Gale, 1989).

Role play as an education method emerged from this background. Role play involves the setting up of an imagined and possible situation, acting out that situation and learning from the drama. After a role play, a period of reflection is necessary, followed by feedback from other participants in order that new learning can be absorbed from the drama.

The first stage of a successful role-play, 'setting the scene', consists of inviting a number of participants to play out a scene, either from their own past or one they are likely to encounter in the future. Scenes replayed from the past are useful in that the role play allows further reflection on those past situations. Anticipated scenes, on the other hand, allow for the rehearsal of new behaviour.

Once the 'players' have been selected, scenery and props of a simple sort should be used to create the invoked scene, for example, tables and chairs, suitably arranged. Once scenery has been set and roles cast, the role play can begin. The facilitator acts as 'director' and helps the actors to fully exploit their roles. Occasionally the facilitator may stop the role play and allow characters to slow down their acting or take time out to consider how best to play the next part of the scene.

When the scene has been played out to the satisfaction of the players, the facilitator asks the players to reflect on their performances and those of their colleagues. An appropriate feedback order is as follows:

- The principal actor self-reports on his or her performance.
- The supporting actors offer the principal actor feedback on their performance.
- The audience offers the principal actor feedback on their performance.
- Those three stages are repeated for all the other actors.
- The audience then evaluates all the actors' performances and offers them feedback.

Following such feedback (which takes considerable time and should not be hurried), the role play can be re-run and new learning, gained from the feedback, can be incorporated into the new performance.

Role play is particularly useful for teaching and learning in the following domains of interpersonal skills training:

- counselling skills training (Nelson-Jones, 1981; Burnard, 1989b)
- group facilitation training (Heron, 1989b)
- assertiveness training (Alberti and Emmons, 1982; Bond, 1987)
- social skills rehearsal (Ellis and Whittington, 1981).

Apart from the use of role play in the development of interpersonal skills, it may also be used as an aid to developing empathy; to rehearse initial practitioner/client meetings; to develop interview skills; to practise public speaking or the delivery of seminar papers and as a problem-solving activity. In this later context, a problem situation is acted out with a variety of possible 'solutions'. The actors and the audience decide which solution feels best after they have completed the various role plays.

Figure 2.4 offers a simple map of the role play that can be used for setting up role plays in a variety of educational situations. Some people love role play: some hate it. As with other activities in this field, participation should never be forced and only those people who *want* to take part should do so. Much can be learned vicariously by watching others engaged in role play.

Problem-solving

The problem-solving cycle (Figure 2.5) is very similar to the nursing process of the research cycle. It offers a practical and logical sequence of events for solving personal, nursing or management problems. Its use is vital as part of the process of developing the critical thinking discussed above. Such a cycle can be used by individuals on their own or by groups and is experiential in that once again it draws upon direct personal experience. It combines, too, both the learning *through* and learning *from* aspects of experiential learning. Learning through experience comes as a

Stage One: Setting the scene; a situation or plot is decided upon.

Stage Two: Actors are selected from the group to play out various roles. Outline 'scripts' are established.

Stage Three: The role play is carried out.

Stage Four: Actors in the role play evaluate their own performances and share what they have learned with the audience.

Stage Five: The audience evaluates the performances of the actors and shares what they have learned.

Stage Six: The actors are debriefed and encouraged to return to their normal selves through the use of distracting questions such as 'Can you tell me what you are planning to do this afternoon' or 'Describe the room we are sitting in'.

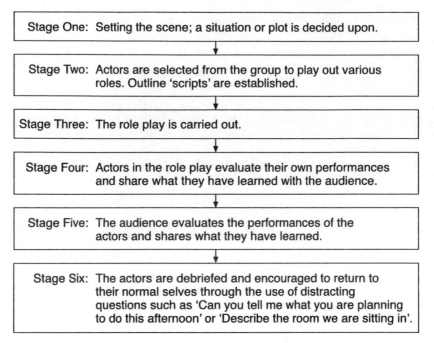

Figure 2.4   A simple map of role play

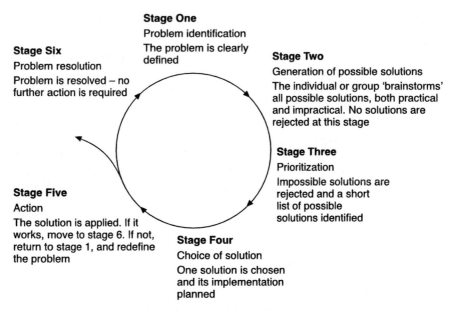

Stage One
Problem identification
The problem is clearly defined

Stage Two
Generation of possible solutions
The individual or group 'brainstorms' all possible solutions, both practical and impractical. No solutions are rejected at this stage

Stage Three
Prioritization
Impossible solutions are rejected and a short list of possible solutions identified

Stage Four
Choice of solution
One solution is chosen and its implementation planned

Stage Five
Action
The solution is applied. If it works, move to stage 6. If not, return to stage 1, and redefine the problem

Stage Six
Problem resolution
Problem is resolved – no further action is required

Figure 2.5   A problem-solving cycle

result of using the cycle itself and learning from experience during the 'brainstorming' phase when solutions are drawn from past experiences of problems. The term 'brainstorming' refers to the free and spontaneous generation of ideas without any attempt at censoring or filtering out less practical ideas.

The basic method of brainstorming may be described as follows. The learning group is encouraged to consider a particular topic and to call out words that they associate with it. These words are then collated on to either a black or white board or onto a series of flip-chart sheets. If the sheets are used they can be hung around the room to form a series of posters that serve as memory aids. During this initial process of calling out of associations, the group is encouraged not to discount any association – often the more bizarre ones can lead to creative thinking (Koberg and Bagnall, 1981).

This process of encouraging associations can be a short one, taking, perhaps, up to 5 or 10 minutes, or it can evolve into a lengthy session of up to 40 minutes, as a means of investigating a topic in depth. The noting down of associations in this way can be an end in itself. The activity can lead into a discussion or a more formal lesson. In this sense, brainstorming is used as a warm-up activity to encourage initial thought about a topic.

The problem-solving cycle has many applications in the nursing field. In nurse education it may be used as a learning aid and it may also be useful as a revision aid when preparing for examinations. In the practical nursing situation it may help to identify novel ways of solving nursing problems. Nurses may also find it helpful in solving personal problems: difficulties with relationships, career changes, financial difficulties and so forth.

The experiential learning approach: an overview

In the foregoing pages, a variety of approaches to the concept of experiential learning have been discussed. They vary in their focus and in their intention. What they all have in common is their use of human experience as the basis of learning. In the experiential learning model, learning is not a process by which facts are 'tacked on' to the person, nor is the person 'filled with knowledge'. The experiential approach acknowledges the broad and vital nature of human experience and sees it as the potential medium for fruitful learning. Figure 2.6 shows the diversity of the approach by drawing together the examples discussed so far. It will be noted, too, that the aspects of experiential learning outlined in the diagram and in the text cover all the aspects of self-awareness discussed in the previous chapter: thinking, feeling, sensing, intuiting and body experience.

Experiential learning and the nurse

The three elements that go to make up the concept of experiential learning are personal experience, reflection and the transformation of knowledge. There are also at least three domains in which the nurse can benefit from

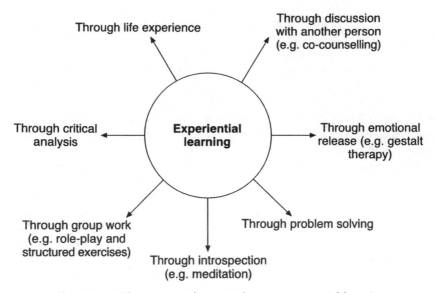

Figure 2.6   The variety of approaches to experiential learning

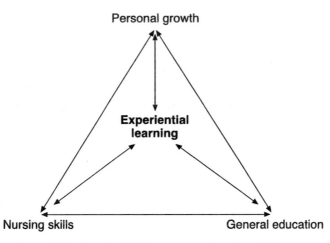

Figure 2.7   Experiential learning methods and the nurse

the experiential learning approach. These are personal growth, in general education and for the development of nursing skills (Figure 2.7).

Experiential learning enhances personal growth by enabling us to develop self-awareness and to understand ourselves better. Through introspection and by receiving feedback from others we can begin to piece together more and more of the separate parts that go to make up the complex whole that we are. Second, through methods such as group work we can explore our relationship with others. As nursing is so particularly a relationship concerned with caring for others (Morrison, 1989), it is crucial that we understand both ourselves and our abilities and weaknesses in dealing with others. Once again, we cannot begin to understand those two facets until we map out the territory, until we become aware of what we are like and how we relate to others. Armed with such awareness we are better prepared to modify our interpersonal behaviour as we see fit.

The critical ability developed through questioning our experience can help in the domain of general education. If nursing is to continue to become a research-based profession it is vital that we arm ourselves with the necessary tools for questioning and challenging what we see and what we, ourselves, do. The reflective and critical aspects of experiential learning can help here.

Third, experiential learning methods are particularly valuable in learning nursing skills, particularly the interpersonal, human skills. Thus our ability to open conversations with others comes through the *experience* of opening conversations. The skills of helping someone who is in tears develops through the *experience* of talking to someone who is crying. Conversely, being the partner of someone who is practising and developing such skills further develops our ability to relate to others. Experiential training techniques combine practice with personal experience: the chance to develop interpersonal skills through attention to the self and to others.

Next, attention is turned to the combination of experiential learning and andragogy and finally, to nurse educators' perceptions of experiential learning.

Curriculum planning in nurse education: experiential learning and andragogy

Andragogy, a term associated with Malcolm Knowles (Knowles, 1978, 1980, 1984) although used before his time, is one employed to differentiate the theory and practice of adult education from pedagogy – the theory and practice of the education of children. Knowles claimed that adults differed in some fundamental ways from children and, therefore, required a different educational system. Such a system included the ideas that:

- Adult education should be grounded in the participants' wealth of prior experience.
- Adults need to be able to apply what they learn.
- Adult education should be an active rather than a passive process.

All of these ideas have much in common with the concept of experiential learning described here. Out of these ideas, Knowles drew up a method of conducting adult education sessions.

One objection that may be raised about Knowles's theory is that the ideas identified above may be applicable, also, to children. If this is the case, it is difficult to see how he can argue for a discrete theory of adult education based on these principles. Knowles acknowledges this problem and, in later writing, tends to describe andragogy as an attitude towards education rather than as being a discreet theory of adult education. This argument and others relating to andragogy have been well described by Jarvis (1983, 1984) and Brookfield (1987).

Andragogy has much in common with the student-centred learning approach of the late Carl Rogers (1983). This is not surprising as both Knowles and Rogers were influenced, through their respective professors of education, by John Dewey, the pragmatist and philosopher of education (Dewey, 1966, 1971; Kirschenbaum, 1979). It also has much in common with many of the approaches to experiential learning, emphasizing, as they do, the centrality of personal experience and subjective interpretation.

How, then, may aspects of experiential learning and andragogy usefully be combined in nurse education? Such a combination needs to take into account certain basic principles such as negotiation, the importance of personal experience and the use of self and peer assessment. What must also be borne in mind, however, is that learner nurses and nurse educators have to work to a prescribed syllabus of training laid down by the English and Welsh National Boards even if such syllabi are *interpreted* by individual schools and colleges. This fact makes nurse education somewhat different to many of the experiential learning training workshops at which all of the content may arise out of participants' needs and wants. Many nurse educators may encounter problems in translating workshop experience into practice because of this fact. Also, there is a large difference between using experiential learning methods in a 2-day to 1-week training workshop and using them on a regular basis throughout a 3-year programme.

Figure 2.8 offers a tentative cycle which acknowledges both the principles of andragogy and the principles of experiential learning, as outlined in this chapter.

In Stage One, two things happen. First, the students identify their own learning needs through direction from the tutor and in line with the 'learning contract' approach described by Knowles (1975). Second, the tutor identifies certain learning needs out of the prescribed syllabus. The students can draw from their previous ward experience, here, and may find a 'brainstorming' session a useful means of generating topics.

Thus, in Stage Two, a timetable is negotiated. It will consist of the two elements described above and may be divided into a 'theory' element and a 'skills' element. The skills element may include both practical nursing skills and interpersonal skills, as appropriate. Again, it will be remembered that the content of this theory and skills mix will arise jointly out of the expressed needs of the students and the suggested ideas of the nurse tutor.

The theory element may then be learned using a whole range of educational approaches, including the traditional ones of lecture and seminar, as required. However, for the skills element, it is recommended that the experiential learning cycle be followed.

The cycle, briefly outlined here, incorporates the student-centred, negotiating approach of andragogy with the accent on personal experience and self and peer evaluation of experiential learning. It also acknowledges

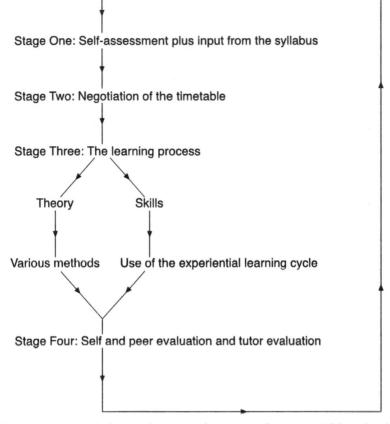

Figure 2.8 A cycle for combining andragogy and experiential learning in nurse education

that learner nurses need to work to a syllabus and that nurse educators can contribute much to effectively planning a course of study around such a syllabus. In this cycle, 'negotiation' means just that – the programme emerges out of the experience and knowledge of both students and tutors.

The approach offers a balance between what Heron (1986) calls 'following' and 'leading'. Following involves taking the lead from the students, using their experience and ideas. Leading, on the other hand, means making suggestions and using structure to help the students. Together, these methods can ensure balance and symmetry in the nurse education programme. If the programme involves too much 'following' or is too student-directed in its methods, it will be unbalanced. On the other hand, if it involves too much 'leading' or is too teacher-directed in its methods, it will also be unbalanced.

Having said this, the attitude towards nurse education should always remain student-centred. The issue is not whether or not the tutor or the student should serve as the focal point of the educational process but the means by which the student's educational needs are identified and satisfied. In this sense, then, the focus remains the student.

Conclusion

This chapter has explored the concept of experiential learning from a variety of points of view. It started by noting the variety of definitions that have been used in the literature. It then explored aspects of the concept that seem common to *all* approaches to experiential learning. Humanistic and other themes common in the experiential learning approach were discussed and practical issues explored. In the chapters that follow, those themes are translated into practice through a discussion of reflection as an experiential learning method, and the offering of the findings of a research project and of ranges of experiential learning activities for the development of counselling and group skills. Self-awareness continues as a prerequisite of all skilful human intervention.

In closing this chapter, it is important to consider the question of training for experiential learning facilitation. David Boud sums up the problems in this area well:

> One of the questions that arises is how sophisticated should training be? Too often those working in experiential education are simply doing what they have picked up as an adjunct to their normal work. They have learned from experience but their experience is limited. There is little training available and, sometimes, desired. However, unless we are challenged to move beyond our existing practices then experiential education will remain forever peripheral to mainstream education and promise more than it can deliver. (Boud, 1989)

Boud was not writing, particularly, about nurse educators and nurse education. But he might have been. As we shall see in the chapter about research, many nurse teachers simply 'pick up' experiential learning methods as they go about their work. There may be a case for incorporating more formal training into teacher training curricula. This has begun to happen but – given the centrality of practical experience in nursing – more work needs to be done to ensure that *all* nurse teachers can help students make the best use of their experience.

Recommended reading

Areglad, R.J., Bradley, R.C. and Lane, P.S. (1996) *Learning for Life: Creating Classrooms for Self-Directed Learning*. London, Sage.

Costa, A.L and Liebmann, R.M. (1997) *Supporting the Spirit of Learning: When Process Is Content*. London, Sage.

Nagel, N.C. (1996) *Learning Through Real-World Problem Solving: The Power of Integrative Teaching*. London, Sage.

Nicklin, P.J. and Kenworthy, N. (2000) *Teaching and Assessing in Nursing Practice: An Experiential Approach*, 3rd edn. London, Harcourt Brace.

Rabow, J., Charness, M., Kipperman, J. and Vasile, S. (1994) *Learning through Discussion*, 3rd edn. London, Sage.

3

Reflection as Experiential Learning

One of the aims of what might be described as the academic educational philosophy (arising, originally, out of Project 2000) was the development of the *reflective practitioner*. The notion of reflective practice is usually linked to the work of Donald Schon (1983) but clearly relates also to educational ideas prior to his writings (Freire, 1972; Wirth, 1979; Mezirow, 1981). Reflection, as an educational tool, has also been advocated by Heron (1973), who described it in terms of 'noticing' or becoming aware of what you are doing, as you are doing it. In the psychiatric nursing field, early papers (Smoyak and Rouslin, 1982) describe the *conscious use of the self* as a therapeutic enterprise. The notion involved consciously using certain personal skills in everyday psychiatric nursing practice and thus acting as a reflective practitioner. In the previous chapter, the idea of learning *through* and *from* experience as part of an experiential learning cycle was referred to – a process which, again involves the practitioner in being aware of his or her own psychological, cognitive and behaviour state. Indeed, reflection may even be described as a particular state of consciousness: consciousness or awareness of events, in the present time and as they happen, with the 'doer' fully aware of his or her intentions as well as his or her actions.

Jarvis (1992) argued that reflective practice was an essential part of nursing as a professional activity. He makes the point that although nursing tends to be a highly structured and ritualized activity, mentors and supervisors can help neophyte nurses to develop reflective skills. He also suggests that reflective practice can also help nurses to 'grow' both professionally and personally. One of the distinctive features of reflection, is, perhaps, that it is *idiosyncratic*: no two people's reflections are likely to be the same. This subjective learning process can act as a foil and a contrast to the more formal, lecture-based learning sessions that are now offered in many colleges of nursing.

Reflection has its roots in both experiential learning (indeed, it forms the second stage of the experiential learning cycle as we noted in Chapter 1) and in the work of John Dewey. Dewey, in turn, is often cited as one of the philosophers who contributed, considerably, to experiential learning theory. He defined *reflective thought* as follows:

> Active, persistent, and careful consideration of any belief or supposed form of knowledge in the light of the grounds that support it and further conclusions to

which it leads ... it includes a conscious and voluntary effort to establish belief upon a firm basis of evidence and rationality. (Dewey, 1933)

Again, this is very similar to the concept of experiential learning itself. Dewey is arguing that reflection is a *voluntary* and intentional action. He is suggesting that the person who does the reflecting remains open to the possibility of changing – both in terms of beliefs and knowledge and – presumably – as a person. It is interesting to note, too, that he suggests that the person doing the reflection looks for *evidence* to support the new way of thinking and appeals to *rationality*. These two factors lead us to a similar position to that described in Chapter 1 under the heading of *critical thinking*.

Boyd and Fales (1983) follow Dewey fairly closely when they define reflection as follows:

The process of internally examining and exploring an issue of concern, triggered by an experience which creates and clarifies meaning in terms of self, and which results in a changed conceptual perspective.

On the other hand, Murphy and Atkins (1994), writing specifically from a nursing point of view, offer the following, pithy observation:

Reflection is initiated by an awareness of uncomfortable feelings and thoughts which arise from a realization that the knowledge one was applying in a situation was not itself sufficient to explain what was happening in that unique situation.

Murphy and Atkins point to a critical point in anyone's thought processes: the point at which we realize that those theories and beliefs we have held up to now are no longer completely viable: what we took for granted is no longer enough. This puzzling and uncomfortable situation is not to everyone's liking and – presumably – some people merely rationalize their situation or try to make the situation they find themselves in fit *their* beliefs. In other words, they work things around until the world fits *their* picture of it. Referring to the uncomfortable nature of reflection and the difficulty of staying open to it, Saylor (1990) writes this:

I've been thinking recently about how difficult it is to be reflective ... I often feel like I don't have enough time to step back and evaluate how effective I am. By the time I finish one day, I usually feel like there is still next day's mountain to climb ... Another thing about reflection – it's hard. It's hard because one must analyse what's transpired and to some degree, make a value judgement about it. And if the reflection is honest, it can mean that I may have to alter my style or completely chuck something that I have worked hard to develop.

Reflection, then, means living with uncertainty and remaining open to the distinct possibility of being wrong. The adult educator Stephen Brookfield confirms the 'uncomfortable' nature of reflection and the triggers that cause it:

there is always some 'trigger' for reflection. Some unexpected happening prompts a sense of inner discomfort and perplexity. (Brookfield, 1987)

Part of the 'trick' of reflection, then, is staying open to it and *remembering* to reflect. This sort of reflection takes practice and discipline. It is often easier and 'safer' *not* to reflect for, by not doing so, we are not forced to face a revision of our ideas and practices. Palmer, Burns and Bulman (1994) offer a series of essays about the theoretical and practical issues surrounding the use of reflection in nursing practice.

In summary, Kemmis (1985) offers a useful summary of what he describes as the 'nature of reflection':

1. Reflection is not biologically or psychologically determined, nor is it 'pure thought'; it expresses an orientation to action and concerns the relationship between thought and action in the real historical situations in which we find ourselves.
2. Reflection is not the individualistic working of the mind as either mechanism or speculation; it presumes and prefigures social relationships.
3. Reflection is not value-free or value-neutral; it expresses and serves particular human, social, cultural and political interests.
4. Reflection is not indifferent or passive about the social order, nor does it merely extend agreed social values; it actively reproduces or transforms the ideological practices which are at the basis of the social order.
5. Reflection is not a mechanical process, nor is it a purely creative exercise in the construction of new ideas; it is a practice which expresses our power to reconstitute social life by the way we participate in communication, decision-making and social action.

Kemmis brings a political, cultural and social edge to the debate about reflection. He is arguing that reflection is not something that a single person does in isolation but that any reflection is contextual. The fact that we are in a particular social, political and cultural context means that our *personal* reflections are also a comment on our shared situation. Given the social and cultural dimension in which nursing exists, and given that fact that nursing is a 'social' occupation in the sense that we are always nursing other people, these points are useful in considering how to *apply* the concept of reflection both in nursing education and in the practice setting. Also, *shared* reflection can lead not only to individual change but also to group change. In reflecting on our knowledge and practice in the company of others we come to modify our ideas and beliefs about the world in a way that we never could if we were alone. Consider, for a moment, the difference between studying alone and studying in a group. One of the things that marks out group study as an effective approach to learning is that it offers the opportunity of 'live', active and spontaneous debate: new learning really *is* new, in that such a debate has never before taken place in *quite* the way it is at this time and in this place. In a group, our beliefs and thought processes are being challenged by others and, contrariwise, *their* beliefs and thought processes are also being challenged. This form of reflection, then, involves *reciprocity*: in group reflection, we are 'fellow travellers' in the learning process. Also, we can never anticipate where the journey will take us or where it will end.

Powell (1989) developed the reflective diary or journal both as a means of enabling students to reflect on their learning processes and as a way of recording new learning. Lyte and Thompson (1990) described the use of such reflective diaries as the means of evaluation and renegotiation of clinical learning objectives in a post-basic mental health nursing course. They suggested that diaries may fulfil the following aims:

- facilitate the development of a problem-solving practitioner who can assess various care options in response to differing needs and evaluate his or her interventions effectively;
- encourage the efficient use of independent learning by stimulating motivation to set his or her own learning objectives;
- assist in the reconciliation of theory-practice issues through exploration of applied theory to practice;
- assist in the development of the student's personal growth through increased self-awareness in relation to patient and colleague interactions;
- assist in the student's professional growth by identifying skills-based learning needs and enabling contracts of learning to be formulated between tutorial or clinical staff in conjunction with established theoretical and clinical objectives; function as an integrated part of the formative assessment process enabling feedback of information to both the teacher and student.

Here we see a coming together of all of the stages of Kolb's experiential learning cycle in nursing practice. The students in Lyte and Thompson's study were subject to their experience of their clinical placements and college learning. Those students then reflected on what had happened to them and on what they had learned and recorded those reflections in their diaries. The diaries then formed the basis of both informing future clinical practice and of identifying new learning objectives.

Nurse educators' views of reflection and reflective practice

A qualitative study was carried out to explore nurse teachers' perceptions of reflection. Given the fact that reflection is a relatively 'new' educational approach, it was decided to invite a range of nurse teachers to describe their views on the topic.

The sample was a purposive one (May, 1993). Purposive sampling is a non-probability sampling method and one in which the respondents are chosen for the study according to the likelihood of their being able to talk on the topic in hand. If a researcher is exploring reflection with nurse educators then it is appropriate that 'nurse educators' become the population from which that sample is drawn.

LoBiondo-Wood and Haber (1994) confirm that sample sizes in qualitative studies tend to be small and suggest that interviewing should continue until 'data saturation' has occurred – that is, until no 'new' ideas or thoughts are identified by the respondents. In this study, this occurred by the eighth interview and the research continued until 12 interviews had been completed.

The 12 nurse educators, from a range of institutions, were interviewed using a semi-structured interview schedule. The semi structured interview allows the researcher to become an active participant in the interview while, at the same time, making sure that certain key areas are discussed (Gilbert, 1993).

All the interviews were taped and each interview lasted between 30 minutes and 1 hour. The interviews were transcribed and then content-analysed. Content analysis – of the sort used here – involves identifying a range of themes within the transcripts and then reordering the text to reflect those themes (Sapsford and Abbott, 1992; May, 1993). The aim of the analysis was to account for all of the different points of view discussed by the respondents and to try to avoid 'researcher bias'. An attempt was made to cut away 'dross' (Field and Morse, 1985) – those aspects of the text that did not bear, directly, on the research topic. The notion of 'dross' does, of course, beg the question of what might *count* as dross and here the researcher has to make fairly autocratic decisions about what to leave in the account of the study and what to leave out.

The findings are described here under a series of headings and are interspersed with commentary about the various points that arose.

Reflection in nurse education

Many of the respondents defined reflection in much the same way as definitions are found in the literature (Schon, 1983; Atkins and Murphy, 1993). They included descriptions of reflection as involving looking back over clinical practice and thinking about what they did as nurses during that period of practice. Examples of typical responses are as follows.

> It is the process of auditing aspects of caring that nurses do. As a professional that is still involved clinically with using reflection in my practice, it is very much looking at what I do, why I do it and how it works.

> It is helping students to look at their practice in a manner that is designed to make the person explore and use what they have found that is good and understand, perhaps, what was difficult or problematic and that they could put into their ongoing practice.

> It is an opportunity to stand back, to take stock, to look at a particular incident and to look at what has happened in a professional way.

> It is the opportunity to say 'Well, how did I perform and what could I have changed. What could I have done that was different? What would I do if it happens again?'

It will be noted that the first respondent, above, noted the importance of her link with *clinical practice* as a nurse educator. Some respondents linked the use of reflection to the literature and made it a more 'formal' learning activity – perhaps more in keeping with the literature that describes *experiential* learning as described in the previous chapter. For example, one respondent said:

> I understand it is a technique used to encourage students to reflect on practice and to read the literature surrounding that practice so that they become more informed.

This respondent is suggesting that reflection may lead to a desire to learn more – a point discussed by Wlodkowski (1985) in his discussion of motivation in adult learning. The main point, in this category, however, was the degree of *similarity* between respondents in the way that reflection was defined.

Reflective practice in nurse education

Sometimes a distinction was made between reflection and reflective practice, although as the respondents talked often these two concepts merged into one. For instance, one respondent said:

> Actually, I am not clear in my own mind that there is a distinction made by nurses between reflection and reflective practice.

Other respondents talked about the idea of reflective practice as part of the process of nursing and as an important aspect of nurse education.

> [Reflective practice] is thinking about practice during practice: thinking about practice after practice in relation to various aspects of the process of nursing.

> It means thinking about your practice, about your relationship with others and about the way you feel about, say, performing certain tasks. Really in a sense it is becoming more self-aware of your own practice.

Clearly the above respondent had linked reflective practice and the more general idea of self-awareness, although the issue was not elaborated on by the respondent nor taken up by the interviewer. Another respondent linked reflective practice to the idea of the nurse's role and suggested that:

> reflective practice is one way, you know, after events, of trying to break down what happened and thinking about what role you had in them and what you did and why you did certain things and trying to decide 'was that the right thing to do?', 'did it work, was it effective or perhaps I should have done something else?'

Another respondent thought that reflective practice was perhaps just a new name for something that was already being done – a point echoed by others and reported in another section of this chapter.

> Well, I suppose it is just to do with thinking about what you are doing and learning by previous experience, but under another name.

This respondent again echoes the stages of the experiential learning cycle as described by Kolb (1984), Weil and McGill (1989) and others and discussed in the previous chapter. This respondent's comments seem to echo the concepts underlined by those writers on experiential learning, emphasizing, as they do, the need to link *thinking* about experience with experience *itself*.

Nursing and the use of reflection

Many respondents were excited by the idea of reflective practice and felt that it was a very useful way of helping people to improve the work they did as nurses, for instance one suggested, simply, that:

> You can't do without it!

The point seemed to be that everyone needs to reflect – both in and out of nursing. Other respondents were similarly enthusiastic.

> I think it is an exciting opportunity in a professional way to combine both theory and practice for an improvement in practice.

> It is a good thing that nurses have tended to become reflective. I think that some nurses in the past would 'unpack' the day at the end of the day and talk to their colleagues about things and reflect on actions but I think I have discovered as a teacher that a surprising number of nurses don't or haven't ever re-opened the box once something has gone by and I think that we can only learn from our mistakes and to try to do things better planned in the future.

This respondent is clearly seeing reflective practice as a way of future planning and as a way of enhancing future practice. He is also critical of a more traditional nurse who might not stop and think about what they did in practice. However not all respondents were equally enthusiastic. One respondent, for example, had ambiguous feelings about the value of reflective practice in nursing.

> I feel it can be a mixed blessing. I am a bit concerned because it seems to have appeared from nowhere. It has obviously got some value but I am concerned that it is seen as a panacea. I think it is very important there should be certain strategies and safeguards for the person's personal, intimate emotions. Otherwise, it is an invasion of a person's private views. Thinking about things is good, yes, but in a sense I wonder if reflecting on things is not just a part of being human. It may be too *introspective*. In a way it is possible for you to get *paralysis from analysis* by not looking at what is happening here and now and what might happen in the future but by forever looking back.

This respondent whilst acknowledging the value of reflection also notes that too pointed a reflective session might encroach on the person's personal life. It was felt by this respondent to be really important that we respect that people have a choice about the things they talk about and the feelings they express. It is vital that no one feels under pressure to reflect in company about those things they would prefer to keep private. One respondent discussed an experience in a College of Nursing in which student's 'private' reflective journals had been discussed, openly, in the staff room.

On a similar but different theme another respondent had this to say:

> I've seen and experienced words like reflection before which have become a hobby horse or a bandwagon or an academic exercise and I have really not sufficiently thought through what was clearly expressed by educators and practitioners. Nurses have developed a very sophisticated oral culture and nurses are incredibly clever and gifted at oral expression, oral argument

and so on but are notoriously weak at writing down their experiences and I think that if reflection can help us do that then we are moving nursing forward.

Some respondents described what could happen if you don't encourage nurses to reflect. For example, one respondent had this to say:

I think that if you don't reflect, if you cannot encourage reflection or debriefing or whatever you call it, if you don't encourage nurses to record incidents or situations and items from their practice and to think about those and to share them, to tell their stories and to examine those stories then nursing will stagnate. It will regress and it will really have increasing problems in demonstrating that it has any value in the future.

This was a particularly strong response about what might happen if reflection didn't occur and raises the rather odd question of whether or not there could be any human situation in which *no* reflection occurred at all. As we have noted, some respondents felt that reflection was an automatic, human process that 'naturally' occurred.

Other respondents were unsure about how reflection 'worked' but were convinced from a pragmatic point of view that it was a useful concept. For example, one said:

I don't know quite how it works but all I can see is that when somebody's got it and I can see when they haven't got it. You know it's quite obvious when you work with them for a couple of hours and I am very, very positive about it. I think it's absolutely crucial.

What is interesting about this response is that the respondent seems to indicate an intuitive element to the reflective process. She acknowledged that she could identify another person who 'had it' and also those that did not. This point might usefully have been explored further. The same respondent went on to make very positive statements about reflective practice in nursing.

Well, I'm really into it actually in a big way and it is not because of what I have read it is because of the way I have learnt it in practice. So it comes very much from my work area and the way that I have learnt from things. It was only afterwards that I went to the books and the journals and read about reflection and models of reflection and really saw that this had become formalized and that was why I became really keen on it because I realized that it was something I was doing automatically in my work.

This is an interesting example of *reflection in practice*. This respondent is saying that she noticed that she was reflecting on her practice as she worked in clinical settings. She then went to the literature and made the link between her own professional experience and what had been written in the books and the journals. This response is also an illustration of *how* enthusiastic some educators can be about reflection – a point discussed at length in an analysis of the teaching of reflection by Reid (1993).

Despite generally positive feelings about reflective practice a few respondents had negative comments about it, and one that seems to summarize some of these feelings is as follows:

I don't see that it has any use in nursing at all. There are other learning theories that would be much, much more suited but aren't applied.

However, in retrospect, the interviewee did not elaborate on what those 'other learning theories' might have been, nor did the researcher explore with her whether or not reflective practice was being counted as a formal learning theory.

The advantages of being a reflective practitioner

Many advantages were cited by respondents although most of them related to improvement of clinical practice. For example one respondent said:

I think that it makes you a more confident practitioner and a more competent practitioner. It makes you a more sensitive practitioner as well. It gives you an opportunity to look at your practice and to try to improve on it.

Another respondent linked it directly to cognitive processes (and directly to patient care) when he suggested that:

I think the benefits are that people become more thoughtful, they intellectualize the process of nursing more and ultimately it is for the betterment of the client.

Yet another respondent linked the use of reflective practice to *quality issues*. Offering a quote that could have been taken directly out of a book on quality assurance (see, for example Munro-Faure *et al.*, 1993), a respondent suggested that 'you are more likely to get it right first time, next time'. There is some ambiguity in the above phrase. If you are going to get it right first time, then there isn't a next time!

Other respondents identified the fact that reflection actually changed the way in which you felt about the world. One respondent talked about how it could make nurses less certain about the situation in which they found themselves:

I think that it enables you to realize that nothing is certain and there is no right answer. It gives a nuance – a balance. It means that decisions are being made through evaluating the information given at the time. I think that being a reflective practitioner is thinking about things as you are doing them or once they are done. After a long time it may be useful. The best thing to realize is that there is a lot of uncertainty in the decision-making process and in practice. The nurse's role is to live with uncertainty and to try to make the best decisions even with that uncertainty.

The respondent echoes a number of writers on adult education who have stressed the need for adults to adopt a *critical* viewpoint and to resist any attempt to find 'the' answer to real life issues (Claxton, 1984; Brookfield, 1986, 1987). Another respondent offered the suggestion that reflection could also be an uncomfortable process in as much as it forced change.

I think that reflection is painful because what it does is it actually challenges and brings to the fore the whole idea of change. In a sense reflection can speed up change and change is never easy, it is never comfortable and sometimes it can be very frustrating.

Overall though the responses were positive about the idea of reflective practice in nursing. Many respondents described how the reflective approach could enhance patient care – although *specific* examples of how that enhancement could take place were not offered.

I think the advantages are that we get a more thoughtful, purposeful, systematic approach to nursing using a reflective approach.

Well I think it helps you develop your own practice. It helps you to enquire, so for instance you may be able to reflect on something that has happened and answer all the questions that you have – your own questions – but you might not so then you go to the library, a book or a journal to find out. Or you might ask somebody else who you think might know. So I think from your knowledge and enquiry it can help you to change the way you feel about your practice.

The disadvantages of being a reflective practitioner

For some respondents there was a sense that we'd 'been here before'. One respondent summed this up by suggesting that:

probably the biggest difficulty is the assumption that it may take a long time to do and that in fact we might be doing it already anyway.

Others had specific points that they wanted to make about the disadvantages of reflective practice. One for example worried about the structure that it brought to bear:

Any structure that you use as a guide to reflection can perhaps hinder rather than allow freedom, but it is difficult to get the balance right, because you need a framework in order to do it. I think that probably one of the major disadvantages is that it is part of the national profile.

The last comment about the national profile referred to the fact that national boards for nursing had incorporated the idea of reflective practice very readily into their documents regarding nurse education. It was often noticed in passing that the national boards tended to adopt what might be described as 'popular ideas'. This idea that reflective practice was a fashionable concept was echoed by a number of respondents.

There is a flavour of elitism involved as well, but mainly my concern is dealing with the mumbo-jumbo that is bandied around about reflection. What – to my mind – we are talking about is simply the process of thinking, of reviewing what has happened, what is likely to happen ...

To my mind the disadvantage is that it has been jumped up to make it look like something that is much more sophisticated than it is. Because it is made almost deliberately complex this whole phenomenon is simply muddying the waters; it is making much more of what is just a simple human process and really requires to be one.

I think it is time-consuming and it is probably just a popular exercise at the moment which will lose ground or certainly people will lose interest in it. I think that people have got enough to do without reflecting on every single thing that they do.

Other disadvantages include worries about the students' reactions to personal disclosure and the effect that reflection may have on students:

Oh, there is a touch of navel gazing. The disadvantages are that people become more and more introspective and become more and more anxious about their actions so that they become paralysed by anxiety.

Analysing yourself is not easy and you may dig up lots of things that you may want to leave buried.

I think that it can make nurses as individuals rather introspective. What's past is past and if you are forever looking back you might miss the here and now. Hindsight is an inexact science. Everyone views things from a different perspective. Practice is here and now. Looking back you may get a distorted view. For example, if you are climbing a massive mountain, you may be tired, out of breath, sweating and not really enjoying the experience. But when you have reached the top and you can see the view and you are enjoying the experience you may forget the pain you went through to get to the top – so thinking back on the climb to the top you may get a different perspective on the journey. Is it morally and ethically correct to ask people to reflect on their intimate values? Is that right? What other professionals ask you to reveal your deepest thoughts – has anyone got the right to ask? There is the fear of making the professional deal with the past and not seeing the here and now and looking to the future. What nurses are asked to reveal is deep and significant. At the end of the day I believe that people are selective and tend to choose safe episodes in education and in practice. They tend to choose things from a superficial level. I can see that more trust and safeguards are needed in practice and in education. Effective trust is needed for significant reflection.

This is an important comment on the way in which our perspective on things can change with hindsight. There may be the temptation to believe that when we reflect back on experience we are remembering things as they actually happened. What seems likely is that our recollections are quite different to the flow of events themselves (Claxton, 1984). The question that needs to be raised here is whether or not that matters. Clearly, for the above respondent, the issue was a vital one.

Teaching reflection and reflective practice

Respondents were at times vague about exactly how they taught reflection to students. A number of them referred to a range of experiential learning activities such as group work and a number referred to using explicit models of reflection. However, many more talked in more general terms.

I think that most of my teaching is based probably on looking at critical incidents and looking at reflection and incorporating it into my teaching. So I probably don't teach the theory of it or the framework of it. But I do teach the practical implications of it and we look at critical incidents or scenarios and key concepts.

I tend to use an introductory session as a way of finding out where my students are. I tend to advise them to read certain texts and certain articles. I also use critical incident technique reporting as an assessment strategy for trying to get people more used to reflecting on their actions.

Some respondents seemed doubtful about whether or not they wanted to teach reflection as a formal topic:

I like to think that I don't teach reflection as a subject but I like to feel that personally it is important for people to think about what they learn, what it means for them. I think that I would teach that as a style although I don't teach specifically reflective practice or reflective education.

On the other hand, some respondents were explicit about the types of methods they used to help people to reflect:

I've taught it by setting up workshops, by pairing off students. I make sure that students have a good understanding of reflection and reflective practice by using experiential learning methods.

The point, for a number of respondents, seemed to be that they did not *teach* reflection, in a formal sense, but *modelled* it by demonstrating reflection-in-action to and with their students.

Discussion and conclusion

The findings identified above seem to point to a relative consistency in *defining* reflection but to some disparity about (a) 'how it works' and (b) whether or not it is a 'passing fad'. One the other hand, most of the respondents, with one or two exceptions, expressed very positive feelings about the use and application of reflection in nursing education and in practice. The report, above, also notes some similarities between the reflective process and the experiential learning cycle as described by Kolb (1984) and others. Both processes seem to involve observing a situation, realizing that one is *in* a situation, thinking about it and then making decisions about what to do next. What remains less clear is the degree to which it is necessary or appropriate to *formalize* this sort of process. The respondents in this study appeared to be ambivalent about this issue. As ever, more research needs to be done to clarify the issue – *if*, during the coming years, it is found that the concepts of reflection and of reflective practice remain contemporary. It seems, to this writer, that it is possible (echoing some of the respondents in this study) that reflection is something of a passing interest in nursing. No doubt, though, some of the more important aspects of reflection will become part of the main body of nursing theory and practice while the less important parts fall away.

Reflective activities in nursing

Stein-Parbury (1993) offers the following method of engaging in what she calls *self-reflection* as it relates to thinking about patient care:

1. Describe ... an interaction in terms of what happened. Do not think about why it happened, just what happened between you and the patient.
2. Answer the following questions:
   (a) What did you say that was helpful to the patient?
   (b) What was your intention is saying this?
   (c) How did you know it was helpful?
   (d) What did you say/do that was not helpful to the patient?
   (e) What was your intention in saying this?
   (f) How did you know it was not helpful?
   (g) What could you have said that would have been more helpful?
   (h) What were you feeling during this interaction?
   (i) What do you think the patient was feeling during the interaction?
   (j) How would you have changed this interaction if you could do it again?

One of the problems with this sort of detailed analysis of nurse–patient interaction is that it assumes certain things. First, it assumes that our *recollection* of events matches – at least to some degree – what actually happened. Second, it assumes that there *were* 'unhelpful' things said during any particular intervention. Third, it assumes that the person working through the stages *would* want to change things about that interaction. Apart from those caveats, this sort of systematic reflection on what we do as nurses seems likely to be valuable in helping us to think about what it is we do, why we do it and what the outcomes are. We need to be cautious, however, about assuming too much about our *memory* of various interactions.

In a similar but different approach, Johns (1993a,b) offers the following 'model' for structuring student reflection:

1. **Phenomenon**
   1 Describe the experience
2. **Causal**
   1 What essential factors contributed to this experience?
3. **Context**
   1 What are the significant background factors to this experience?
4. **Reflection**
   1 What was I trying to achieve?
   2 Why did I intervene as I did?
   3 What were the consequences of my actions for:
      myself? the patient/family for the people I work with
   4 How did I feel about this experience when it was happening?
   5 How did the patient feel about it?
   6 How do I know how the patient felt about it?
   7 What factors/knowledge influenced my decisions and actions?

5. **Alternative actions**
   1 What other choices did I have?
   2 What would be the consequences of these other choices?
6. **Learning**
   1 How do I NOW feel about this experience?
   2 Could I have dealt better with the situation?
   3 What have I learned from this experience?

Again, in Johns list there are some questions that *beg* the question. How, for example, can we be sure how we felt about a situation *afterwards*? How might we know what the consequences of any action might be for other people? While there is little doubt that reflecting on our experience might makes us more thoughtful about what we do in the future, we must be careful about too much *attribution*. In other words, we must be careful not to overload our actions with meaning and we must avoid trying to 'best guess' what other people may or may not be thinking about our actions. On the other hand, whether or not we can ever practise 'clean' reflection – in which we do not overlay our own beliefs or values on the past situation – is one more open question.

Enhancing reflection through literature

As we have seen, the aim is to enable nurses to become more reflective in their practice and even in their everyday lives. One means of doing this in nurse education is through the use of *literature*, including extracts from novels, essays and poetry. All three of these media draw on metaphor and in exploring metaphor new insights can be gained. There are a number of ways in which literature can be used and a short list of these might be as follows:

- through encouraging students to read certain novels and poems
- to use selected chapters or passages from novels as the focus for discussion groups
- through encouraging students to read their own choice of literature and then to write essays or discussion papers.

A variety of novels, essays and poems are suitable for this sort of activity and, clearly, they do not necessarily have to have a *nursing* focus. Most literature deals with fundamental human issues: birth, love, relationships, death, emotion and so on. Reflecting on the ways in which these topics are dealt with by particular authors and reflecting on the metaphors used to describe the human condition can enable the student to think more clearly and, perhaps, more sensitively about the work that he or she is engaged in.

If students are offered passages to read or are recommended novels or poems to work through, the following questions can be asked in subsequent discussion groups as the means by which to enhance reflection:

- What did (the particular) metaphor *mean*?
- Why was the author *using* this metaphor?

- How did you feel about this piece of writing?
- What did it say about the human condition?
- What meaning does it have for nursing?

It is difficult to recommend particular literature for particular groups but I have found writing by the following authors to be of value in these sorts of reflective groups (and this is necessarily a short and selective list):

- Primo Levi
- J.D. Salinger
- Jean Paul Sartre
- Scott-Fitzgerald
- Joseph Conrad
- Dylan Thomas
- David Lodge
- Paul Theroux
- T.S. Eliot
- William Shakespeare
- W.H. Auden
- Gerard Manley Hopkins

It must always be borne in mind that one person's favourite novel or poem is not necessarily the next person's. It is important not to *force* reading on others or the point is lost. This is where the selection of *passages* of literature can be useful. Reading a short passage is one thing: reading the whole work – if you don't like the style – is quite another. There is always the possibility of a paradoxical reaction to a recommended book, poem or play: the fact that the lecturer recommends something is enough, for some people, to decide never to read it. Reading literature is a personal experience.

Some lecturers have found that *critical reading* has a place in nursing education programmes. When this approach is used, each student group is encouraged to read a particular work within a week. After that time, a discussion group is convened in which the novel or whatever is discussed critically. This group can be organized along fairly formal lines or can be an unstructured discussion about the novel in question. If structure is used, the following issues can be used to develop that structure:

- What was the main *story* or plot of the novel?
- What can be said about the *characters* in the novel?
- How was the novel *structured*?
- What was the *point* of the novel?
- How did you feel about the novel?
- What lessons, if any, can be learned from it?
- What did you like or dislike about it?

The critical reading group can encourage a number of things. First, the reading of a range of literature that is 'non-nursing', thus encouraging a broader world-view. Second, it can help students to think critically about what they read – both fiction and non-fiction. Third, it can encourage reflective ability through being stimulated to think about a range of human situations.

Other reflective methods

Two other applications of reflection – as part of the experiential learning process – are now described:

- The reflective group
- Reflective evaluation

These are clearly not exhaustive of the ways in which reflection can be used to enhance learning but they do show ways of applying the concept of reflection to concrete practice.

The reflective group

Reflective groups can be organized as part of nurse education and training. They can also be used *in* the community in nursing centres and offices and in health visitor and general practitioner centres. It is probably best that they are run, in the early days, by someone who has some experience of group facilitation (Clarke and Feltham, 1990). Later, the facultative role can be handed over to another group member. In this way, the skills of running groups are learned through the process of being a group member: a particularly effective form of experiential learning (Burnard, 1991).

Ideally, the group should be made up of no more than ten people. Larger groups are possible but they also bring their own problems. Some participants feel inhibited by lots of people in a group. Also, it can be difficult for everyone to contribute when there are many participants. Clearly, the larger the group, the longer it will take to make sure that everyone is heard. Also, a smaller group is usually more intimate and an atmosphere can more easily be developed in which people can be open and frank in their disclosures (Burnard and Morrison, 1992).

A reflective group should not be a 'free for all'. The more structured they are, the more economical use is likely to be made of the time that is available. Groups that have no agenda and no structure can seem aimless. The following guidelines are suggested as signposts for running such a group.

Introductions

First, everyone needs to know who they are sharing the group with. Sometimes, the group will be made up of colleagues or of fellow students. In this case, an introductory activity can be left out. When people do *not* know each other, however, it is useful if each person, in turn, says who they are, where they work and something else about themselves. Such an opening round should be informal but not too prolonged. The aim is to encourage an informal and disclosing atmosphere in the group. However, not all nurses like prolonged 'icebreaking' activities (Cook, 1992) and these may be best avoided.

Describing the activity

Next, participants need a short introduction to the nature of the reflective group. This can be done by the use of a short lecture or discussion about reflective practice and the work of Schon and others. The overall aim is to encourage the participants consciously to learn the skills of reflecting on past and present practice in the community or clinical setting.

Focusing

Group participants may then be asked to focus on a very particular event. For instance, they may be asked to think for a few minutes about their nursing practice in recent weeks and to identify *one* episode of nursing care which they feel they carried out very well. It needs to be stressed that each person needs to think about only one particular incident and that they need to try to remember as much of the detail as possible about that incident: what led up to it, what the patient's needs were, how they planned the episode, how they carried it out and what the consequences were.

The clearer the focus, at this stage, the more specific the activity will become. Also, in focusing in this way, participants are already beginning to learn reflective skills. Once they have been asked to recall an incident in this way and in this detail, they should be given a 5-minute period in which to focus in this way. They may remain in the group or think about the activity away from the group, agreeing to meet back with colleagues after the 5-minute period.

Sharing

Next, participants reassemble in the group and each one, in turn, relates the episode to the rest of the group. This should be done, initially, without any discussion. The individual participant should be encouraged to describe all aspects of the episode as clearly and in as much detail as possible. As a summary, at the end of the description, that individual may be asked to summarize what he or she felt were the *most important aspects of the episode of nursing*. Following this, the participant can invite comments and discussion from the rest of the group. Fellow participants can be asked to comment on the episode of nursing, to offer evaluative remarks and to suggest ways in which the nursing care described could or could not have been improved. There may also be brief discussion about how other people in the group's nursing care compares with that of the colleague who has just spoken. Such discussion should not be prolonged: such discussions can easily degenerate into 'dirty washing' sessions, in which the group merely talks, in a general way, about all the worst and best aspects of nursing. The aim, at all times, should be to keep the focus of attention on the particular episode of nursing under discussion at the time.

Once one participant has described their episode and a discussion has evolved, the facilitator moves on to the next participant who describes the episode that they have considered. The above cycle of events is then continued until everyone in the group has had their say.

Plenary

After each person has discussed the episode they have reflected on, there can be a more general and free-ranging discussion. This can be in two parts. First, there can be a discussion on the issues raised by the individual disclosures. This is a discussion about *content*. The other discussion is one about *process*. Here, the focus of the discussion is 'what was it like to take part in this reflective activity?' A subsidiary question might be 'what are the skills involved in reflection on nursing practice?' In this way, the idea of reflection as a practical adjunct to the nursing process is reinforced and group participants are encouraged to develop the skills that they have begun to use.

A word of caution is in order here. It is not assumed by the writer, nor can it be assumed by the group facilitator that this type of activity will be new to *everyone*. Some people are naturally fairly reflective. Others have periods when they think about what they do and how they do it. For others, however, this may not be the case. Nurses who have been in practice for some time may well find themselves operating on 'automatic pilot' and carrying out their nursing duties without a great deal of reflection. It is this later group that is likely to benefit most from a reflective group although, in the end, almost everyone is likely to benefit.

Moving on

The final stage of the group activity is to move beyond the group, itself, and to carry the skills of reflection into community or clinical nursing practice. This may be achieved more readily if the group reconvenes on a regular basis and the reflective group gradually evolves into a support group. This article has outlined the stages of developing a reflective group for nurses. Reflection is not the whole answer to enhancing nursing care but it can certainly help.

Reflective evaluation

Another method of using reflection in experiential learning is in the form of *reflective evaluation*: a way of helping students to review and make sense of a learning experience.

The aim of reflective evaluation

To evaluate is to place a value on something, to appraise it, to decide on its relative worth. Reflective evaluation invites the student to consider his or her practice, his or her learning or the course of study that he or she has taken part in and to offer a judgement about its relative usefulness or value. This sort of evaluative process works best when it is part of a cycle of events, similar to that illustrated in Figure 3.1. This cycle allows

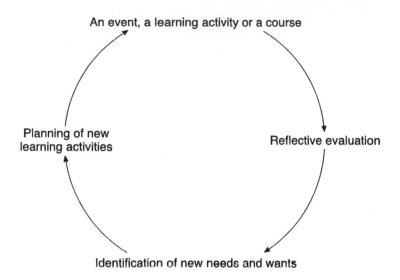

An event, a learning activity or a course

Planning of new
learning activities

Reflective evaluation

Identification of new needs and wants

Figure 3.1   A learning cycle involving reflective evaluation

for reflection on an event, a learning activity or a course of study and then
for the evaluative comments to be fed back into the design process of
management or educational practices. Thus, an educator might use the
reflective evaluation process at the end of a study day or workshop and
then carry the comments generated by it forward into the planning of the
next study day or workshop.

The process

The process of reflective evaluation may be divided into a number of
stages and these are illustrated in Table 3.1.

Stages one and two are those worked through by the facilitator of the
process. He or she invites the group to identify a particular theme,
context, place or course (depending on the context of the activity). For
example, a ward sister may invite students to reflect on their placement in
a particular clinical setting. An educator may ask students to consider a
particular study block in their course of training. In the second stage, the
facilitator encourages further focusing, by asking the group members to
consider a *particular* element in that context. Here, for example, the ward
sister may ask students to think of the *practical nursing experience* that they
gained in a particular clinical setting. Or a nurse educator may invite
students to consider *nursing theory* in a block of study. Thus an *element*,
for the purposes of reflective evaluation, is a small unit of experience,
learning or of a course, which is being considered for evaluation.

Table 3.1 The stages of reflective evaluation

Stage	Activity
Identifying the context	The facilitator helps the group to focus on a particular time period, place or course of study
Locating the element	The focus is sharpened to highlight a particular sort of event, place or session
Reflecting on the element	Each person reflects on the element and makes notes
Publishing and sharing	Each person verbalizes his or her thoughts and feelings on the element, to the group. After the disclosure, the group offer comments and reactions
Discussion	The group discuss any other aspects of the activity and consider the implications of the lessons learned
Feedback	The facilitator draws together the group's comments and prepares, from them, a handout to serve as an *aide-mémoire*
Summary	

Next, participants are asked to reflect on the element and to use the following categories to evaluate it:

- The worst things about the element.
- The best things about the element.
- What could have been different about it.
- What I learned from it.

While participants reflect, they make notes under those headings. Clearly, these headings can be modified and clarified to suit the particular circumstances and context of the activity. The important thing, however, is to make sure that *some* structure is used in this phase of the process. Simple reflection is not enough: for the process to be an evaluative one, some criteria are required against which the participants may make a judgement about the element. This stage of the activity is best carried out in silence and participants may stay in a group or may be allowed to leave the room in which the evaluation is taking place and reassemble as part of a larger group later.

In the next stage, each person in turn is invited to share his or her perceptions and evaluative comments about the element, with the group. This is the 'publishing' sub-stage. Next, he or she can share any other thoughts or feelings that arise out of this plenary session.

Each person, in turn, feeds back his or her comments and reactions and when the person has had his or her turn, that person may invite comments from other people in the group. Such comments should be of the 'prompting' variety. They should be open questions or comments that help the participant to get more out of the experience. The aim is to help the person to expand on his or her reflection. The aim is *not* to generate a general discussion of the topic.

Once each person has disclosed his or her reflective and evaluative comments, the facilitator declares that stage of the activity complete and invokes a more general discussion about the focus of the evaluation. Here, it is useful if the facilitator asks questions that further draw out group members. The use of basic counselling interventions may be helpful here: open questions, reflection of feeling and content, checking for understanding and/or empathy building (Belkin, 1984; Brown and Lent, 1984; Baruth, 1987). Again, the aim is not, generally, to have a discussion *about* the topic in hand but to empower the participants to extract the most out of their experience. During this final stage, the facilitator takes notes and summarizes the gist of the discussion. This is later typed or word processed, duplicated and handed out to each of the participants as an *aide-mémoire*. Such sheets can be organized in such a way so that future evaluative sessions are also recorded using this 'template'. The use of an organized and structured handout encourages participants to file the sheets and to make direct comparisons between current and past evaluation sessions. It is useful, too, if there is a more open, free, discussional session held on an occasional basis during which participants can review the evaluation sessions that they have had to date.

Variations

The cycle of events described in this chapter can be modified in various ways. First, the group undertaking the evaluation can work in pairs, trios or small groups. If pairing is used, each person can take turns in asking evaluative questions of the other. That person's responses are then recorded as notes and these notes are collated by the facilitator, who produces the structured handout at the end of the session. Second, the whole process can be built into a curriculum package and used at key intervals throughout a training session, a workshop or a block of study. In this way, it can be used as both a formative and a summative evaluation method (Rowntree, 1977). Third, the facilitator may elect to invite participants to reflect on the *process* of this evaluation activity. In this way, the whole process of *reflection* can be discussed and analysed. This may help to reinforce the need for participants to reflect, not just during these sorts of structured sessions, but also as part of their everyday work in clinical and community settings. The process of reflection involves certain *skills*, most notably, perhaps, that of *remembering and choosing* to reflect at all. A discussion about reflection, itself, can aid the development of these sorts of skills.

This chapter has offered a structure whereby students, clinicians, managers or any other nursing group can be helped to reflect on their experience and to evaluate that experience. That structure ensures that the *aim* of the activity is clear, as is the *focus* of the reflective session. Finally, the structure described here ensures that written evidence from the evaluation session is collated and fed back to the participants of the evaluation group. Reflection, itself, cannot be an end in itself. Rather, it needs to enable people to draw together their experiences, make sense of them and then to learn from that the process. The recording element can offer a reference point for future evaluative work. Also, if a 'template' or standardized method of recording details of reflective sessions is used, it can also be used to collect data in research projects aimed at exploring the reflective process. At the time of writing, there is a considerable amount *written* about reflection in nursing but relatively little empirical work done in the field. The processes described in this chapter could easily be modified for use in a research study.

Recommended reading

Bolton, G. (2000) *Reflective Practice: Writing and Professional Development*. London, Sage.

Butterworth, T., Faugier, J. and Burnard, P. (1988) *Clinical Supervision and Mentorship in Nursing*, 2nd edn. Cheltenham, Nelson-Thornes.

Jarvis, P. and Gibson, S. (1997) *The Teacher Practitioner and Mentor in Nursing, Midwifery, Health Visiting and the Social Services*, 2nd edn. Cheltenham, Nelson-Thornes.

Light, G. and Cox, R. (2001) *Learning and Teaching in Higher Education: The Reflective Professional*. London, Sage.

4

Experiential Learning Research

The previous chapters have *described* experiential learning in nursing education and practice and *reflection* as an example of experiential learning. This chapter explores some *research* carried out in the broad field of experiential learning as a whole. It is one thing to prescribe a given way of setting up a series of educational encounters and quite another to identify what people make of that prescription. This chapter attempts to answer the question 'What do other people make of experiential learning?'

The main aim of the study described in this chapter was to explore nurse educators' and student nurses' perceptions of experiential learning. No attempt was made to reach a consensus of opinion about the concept but attempts were made to explore any diversity that existed. It was found that a considerable amount of diversity *did* exist and that the 'verdict' on experiential learning was by no means clear.

Methodology

In the study described here, 12 nurse educators and 12 student nurses from various parts of the UK were interviewed using an open-ended, semi-structured approach. The nurse educators were selected on one criterion: that they claimed to use experiential learning methods in their teaching of student nurses. The students were those working in the hospitals and colleges that employed the nurse educators. Later, the findings reported in this chapter were supported and validated by the findings of a questionnaire addressed to a much larger group of nearly 500 nurse educators and students. A more complete and full account of the research study – described in part here – can be found elsewhere (Burnard, 1991).

What the lecturers said

In this section, a report is offered of what the lecturers said about experiential learning. The report comprises verbatim quotations with commentary.

Defining the field

In order to begin to understand how nurse lecturers understood the concept of experiential learning, it was useful to explore their methods of defining terms. In the first section, it is noted how they defined the expression 'experiential learning'. Such definitions were sometimes offered by the lecturers as a response to a question such as 'How would you define experiential learning?' At other times, the definition emerged during the interview as a means of the educator making clear how he or she used that term.

Definitions of experiential learning

Very often, the first attempts an educator made at defining experiential learning proved tautological. A tautology is when something is defined by reference to itself. This leads to circularity: you can only understand the definition if you understand the terms. It also leads to a paradox: if you understand the terms, you don't need a definition! Clear examples of this are as follows:

> I think it is learning from experience ...
> I look upon it as experiencing things ...
> Experiential learning is learning from experience ...

Such definitions were often followed by a more detailed account of how the educator perceived experiential learning. Sometimes, however, there were clearly problems in identifying definitions:

> To me, experiential activity can be non-descriptive in the sense that people allow things to happen and then you can discuss what has happened without ... prediscussion ... I think anything can be turned to an experiential level ...

Many of the nurse lecturers were able to offer examples of experiential learning methods as examples of what they were talking about, whilst finding formal definition of the topic difficult. There may be something artificial in asking people to define terms formally. This idea is supported by some of the lecturers' difficulty in defining experiential learning:

> I think it is difficult to define and I would say that it is concerned with learning that occurs at the present time, in the here-and-now, as they say ...

> I think it is very difficult to define. I can't think of a precise definition of it but I always look on it as actually doing things, experiencing things ...

This difficulty in definition may have been fuelled by another factor. As we have noted in the literature, the term 'experiential learning' is often defined loosely and its definition may vary from author to author in important ways. Another point may be made here. People do not always *define* the things they use or to which they refer. For example, I like music and I listen to it often. I would find it difficult, though, to offer a *definition* of music, even though I am well aware of what it is when I hear it. To insist on definitions may be to miss the point.

Whilst some lecturers defined experiential learning tautologically and others had difficulty in defining it, others used all-encompassing definitions:

> I think any activity could be experiential . . .
> I suppose using the term experiential could involve anything . . .

The problem, here, is that if experiential learning can 'involve anything', the term becomes meaningless – we no longer need an extra term such as 'experiential learning'.

For some, the accent in defining experiential learning was on a time factor. Examples of this time dimension include:

> Learning about things by doing it and also by learning from the past. Ploughing through your previous experience and reflecting on that and then using what you can get from it to go forward.

The idea of learning from the past and relating it to the present is echoed by another respondent who said that 'It's learning from past experience as well as present experience.' This sort of definition has been discussed in Chapter 2 of this book, where a distinction was made between learning from experience (i.e. the past) and learning through experience (i.e. in the present). Another lecturer made a similar point (although adding yet another dimension) when he said: 'So I suppose its learning from experiencing something at the present time. Or maybe even in the future.' This respondent did not dwell upon a theory of HOW a person may learn from experiencing something at the present time, though the notion of forward movement in time is present again. Sometimes, the accent was more definitely on the present.

> It [experiential learning] has to be here-and-now . . . for me . . .

> I would say that it is concerned with learning that occurs at the present time, in the here-and-now, as they say.

This accent on the here-and-now, on present time, is reflected in the humanistic literature on the topic of learning. Humanistic psychology is discussed in more detail in Chapter 2 of this book. In humanistic psychology, the idea seems to be that the present is all that there is – the only place we live is in the present. The practical aspect of learning through present time experience is developed by another of the lecturers:

> So for me [experiential learning] meant things like the clinical placement of student nurses in wards for experience: the practical aspect of nursing that they get in the ward placements, because they were doing things from which they were learning from. But I think the notion of experiential learning extends beyond just the practical 'doing' things. I think it also involves anything that one experiences: (a) practically, from the point of doing things or (b) it is at a psychic level where in conversation with other people, or in contact with other

people, relationships with other people – working experience also comes into it. So, if you like, it is a question of learning from those things which we all do.

This respondent seems to emphasize the practical, utility value of experiential learning as a tool for teaching and learning nursing. He also seems to be hinting at a more personal and interpersonal aspect. This more personal dimension is made more explicit by other lecturers:

[experiential learning is] putting someone in a situation that they may not have been in before so that they can experience what it feels like.

It is that form of learning in which students take an active part, learning from their own experience.

These lecturers appear to be alluding to the idea that experiential learning may be a more personal form of learning than may be the case with other sorts of learning. Sometimes this comparison and contrast with more 'traditional' forms of learning were made more explicit:

I see experiential learning as having less cognitive input, less cognitive assessment and more input from the people who are involved.

I think that there are differences between more traditional ways of doing things and experiential learning. With experiential learning, there is something that can happen and you make use of it. And for me it is more like doing therapy than teaching, because it allows me to utilize what they [the students] bring as people into the situation and you can't pre-plan that.

In summary, it may be noted that a number of the respondents had difficulty in defining the term 'experiential learning' and a number defined it tautologically. Those who could define it tended to talk in terms of: learning in the here-and-now, learning from past or present experience, learning through direct, practical experience or in terms of its involving 'personal learning' of some sort.

Experiential learning methods

If the nurse lecturers sometimes found it difficult to define experiential learning, they had less difficulty in citing examples of what they would call 'experiential learning methods'.

Examples of experiential learning methods could be divided into two groups:

1. experiential learning in the clinical setting; and
2. those activities which nurse lecturers use in colleges of nursing.

The respondents talked more of the second category than of the first. In the 'clinical setting' category, some respondents talked of how they worked in the clinical setting, alongside the students as a means of encouraging and teaching them:

We work with them on the wards quite a lot and you can see then whether they have picked up what you would have expected them to have picked up and learned what you would have expected them to have learned in experiential learning situations.

Another respondent continued the theme of working in the clinical setting as being an example of an experiential learning method:

> another experiential learning method is when the students work on the ward and actually take the temperature of a patient.

In this example, no mention is made of whether the educator sees it as part of her role to work in the clinical setting with the nurses in question. Another educator made explicit the distinction between experiential learning methods as working in the clinical setting and experiential learning methods as methods that are used in the college of nursing:

> I see experiential learning methods as means of helping people to learn through experience and either within the work situation or within a more formal situation – in the classroom.

Here, the classroom setting is perceived as 'more formal', presumably in contrast to the more informal learning that takes place in the clinical setting. The reference could also be an allusion to the tutor's own perceptions of the differences between classroom and clinical learning. Another respondent also made a distinction between the formal and the informal modes:

> In the wards and taking temperatures. That would be an example of an experiential learning method ... [*To the interviewer*] Or do you mean in a formal learning context?

The bridge between particular types of experiential learning methods used in the college of nursing (such as role-play) and 'clinical' types of experiential learning methods was made via experiential learning methods that simulated clinical settings. One educator described such practices graphically:

> If you want a nurse to know what it feels like to be a patient, you stick them on a ward and stick them in bed and let them experience that.

It was notable that the lecturers more frequently described ways in which they *simulated* nursing situations than they described 'real life' clinical situations in which they taught students. The 'bridging' method of experiential learning, through simulation, is also described by another respondent:

> We do some practicals. We, for example, get some of them to act as patients and nurses. And the patients we give various problems to, like telling them they are blind or telling them they are paralysed down one side. And the other students who are 'being nurses' have to feed them and then we talk about what it felt like to actually be fed when you aren't capable of doing this yourself and how the people acting as nurses treat people who are acting as patients.

Here, various elements of Kolb's (1984) experiential learning cycle may be noted in practice. First, the respondent sets up a simulated clinical experience and asks students to adopt roles. Then they act out a particular experience. Afterwards all the 'actors' gather together to reflect on the process and draw out new learning from that reflection.

Experiential learning methods used in the college of nursing

Whilst, as we have seen, a number of the respondents described experiential learning methods as those that involved learning in the clinical setting, others used the term to describe teaching and learning methods they used in the college of nursing. Sometimes, the definition of experiential learning methods was very broad and all-encompassing:

> Experiential learning methods are things like simulation, role play, games, project work, seminar – they are all experiential forms of learning as opposed to where the learner is just a receiver of information.

Here, the respondent appears to be making a distinction between 'information-giving' as a form of teaching and 'something else', which is not so clear, though the suggestion is that a distinction is being made between 'information-giving methods' and 'activities-based' methods. All of the methods that the respondent cites as examples of experiential learning methods involve the learners in some sort of activity (simulation, role play, games, project work and seminar), although it might be argued that the seminar is less of an action technique than the other four.

This accent on activity is developed by another respondent who appears to be grappling with the concept of using personal experience in education:

> Experiential learning methods involve actively participating in something which may involve actual physical activity. Another method would be bringing your own experience, what you have learned from an experience you have had – perhaps into a discussion group from which other people might be able to learn, so everybody is bringing their own experiences ... so perhaps a discussion group would be a form of experiential learning as well ... I think that anything where one takes an active part in it rather than sitting back and being told ... [is an example of an experiential learning method].

What is also notable about this extract is that the respondent appears to be clarifying her thoughts as she speaks. She appears to be discovering examples of experiential learning methods as she talks through the topic. This is evidenced by her saying '... so perhaps a discussion group would be a form of experiential learning as well'. This possible uncertainty over what are and what are not examples of experiential learning methods (or, looked at a different way, this 'thinking on your feet' approach) was evident in other respondents. It is possible that this was another example of *reflection* in practice. The process of being asked to think about examples of experiential learning methods actually helped in the process of *formulating* such examples as the lecturers reflected on the topic.

> ... a seminar in the college ... I think that's probably an experiential learning method, would you say?

> Project work is an experiential approach, I think ... I don't know if everyone would agree with that ...

> ... on the other hand, a demonstration or something in which you take part is experiential, isn't it?

It was notable, too, that these respondents seemed to be seeking *agreement* from the researcher for their definitions.

Role play was frequently cited as an example of an experiential learning method:

> Other examples would be setting up a role play where either the person adopts a different role or their own role and examines how they felt or what happened as a result of that role play.

This respondent distinguishes between two sorts of role-plays: the sort in which the player is asked to adopt a different role from his current one and the sort in which that player remains 'who he is'. A similar distinction is sometimes made in the literature between role play and psychodrama (Goble, 1990).

Typically, in role play, participants are asked to imagine themselves in roles other than their own, whilst in psychodrama, participants act out situations that they have lived through or which they are likely to live through. These varieties of 'role play' are referred to by another respondent:

> The experiential learning method I use most, I guess, is role play. If we are dealing with a specific situation like teaching a group of students basic nursing skills, for example, what I would be doing with that group of students would be enabling them to set up a pseudo situation, a generalization of a clinical situation in a classroom, when they took on, either the roles of the nurse or the roles of the patient.

Another respondent talked of the 'invention' aspect of role play – of the setting up of a contrived situation in order to enhance learning through experience:

> The methods I have seen have been mainly role-play. The role play techniques that I have used were always ones that were constructed. They were sort of directive, I suppose, they were structured. I became aware, through my involvement with a psychodrama therapist of the use of socio-drama and then my techniques became more or less unstructured – unstructured in the sense of non-directive, because I think that we were able to construct a situation that had been experienced by people in the group. And we were able to put them into an action format through drama.

This respondent appears to be making the distinction between role play and psychodrama (or 'sociodrama'), alluded to above. She also appears to be suggesting that psychodrama, or encouraging group members to 'play themselves' and to draw on their own experiences is beneficial and requires less structure and less direction from the facilitator than does role play. Another possibility is that this respondent became more secure or comfortable in using the approach and consequently became less structuring and directing.

Other methods, apart from and sometimes along with, role play were cited as examples of experiential learning methods:

> Things like role play, structured exercises, group work, people working in pairs or threes, exploring concepts and students bringing their own experience to bear in relation to the concept that is being looked at.

> The methods I have used from the very beginning have been exercises, albeit ones of relaxation, meditation, trust type and icebreaking activities as a means of enhancing people's relationships with one another.

Sometimes more traditional teaching methods were cited as examples of experiential learning methods:

> The experience of doing a project, doing the work, is an experience in an educational setting ... project work is an experiential approach, I think.

> It depends how far you want to describe experiential learning methods, I suppose. I mean, you could say that if you listen to a lecture there are experiences you could pick up.

> [*when talking about experiential learning methods*] ... There is also the Open University packs as well, distance learning packages ...

Here, the notion of experiential learning methods has been extended to include project work, lecturing and distance learning, though it is notable that such expansion was the exception rather than the rule. As noted above, when asked for examples of experiential learning methods, most respondents talked of role play, structured group activities and other similar interactive activities.

Finally, in this section, it is interesting to note negative definitions; in other words, to note what the nurse lecturers suggested were not experiential learning methods. The most frequently cited example of what was not an experiential learning method was lecturing:

> Traditionally, I guess, the non-experiential methods of learning would be where the teacher stood in front of the class-room, students traditionally behind desks.

> I would say a lecture is certainly not an experiential learning method.

These, then, are ways in which the nurse lecturers defined experiential learning and experiential learning methods. In the next section it will be useful to explore the lecturers' theories about the experiential approach.

Talking about experiential learning

The nurse lecturers offered a wide range of theories about experiential learning as they talked. In this section, the following categories emerged: theories about the nature of personal experience, theories about student choice in learning, therapy and experiential learning, emotions and experiential learning and, finally, theories about self-awareness. In this section, each of these categories is discussed in turn.

Theories about the nature of personal experience

A number of respondents indicated that they felt that personal experience was an important aspect of experiential learning. That is to say that they suggested that a student should experience something for his or herself rather than only being told about something:

> I don't think that people can understand it to the depth in which they need to just by being told about it [counselling, nursing]. I think there has to be some putting the feet into the water. Even in a role-play situation, that is more likely to enable meaningful insight to occur in the student than if I just tell them something.

This respondent was able to elaborate on this notion of personal experiencing as distinct from only receiving theory:

> If I talk to them about theory, just theory, and make it quite dry, I think they are less likely to learn from that than if I give them clinical experiences. Just me telling them there are steps along the way ... they are unable to integrate for themselves. But I do think that process of integration is more likely with the increased involvement of experiential learning.

The 'increased involvement', for this respondent, appears to be the factor of the student being personally involved in the learning encounter. This involvement in the learning process is stated slightly differently by another respondent:

> If you take basic learners, the majority of their time as a student is experiential learning because they are not in a class, they are on the wards. Nevertheless, it is recognized in nurse education that the learner – by being a nurse – so it is actually the hands-on practice ...

This respondent seems to be suggesting that experiential learning is something to do with 'hands-on practice', of work in the clinical situation as an example of how to learn nursing.

Another aspect of personal involvement as arising out of experiential learning, is described by another respondent:

> I think it would be better if they actually felt it because ... you think you can imagine what it would feel like to role play something but I think until you actually do role play it ... most of the students get caught up in the role they are playing and experience feelings that they may not have realized that they would do.

There are echoes here of the quality referred to in the previous section, that of becoming 'caught up' in what is happening and becoming 'lost' in the role play or activity. What seems to be emerging is a suggested difference between traditional 'learning of facts and theories' and 'learning, personally, through direct involvement'.

Theories about student choice

As we have noted, a number of respondents referred to the personal nature of the learning that takes place under the heading of experiential learning and often described the idiosyncratic and individual nature of students' responses in such learning encounters. This led on to discussions about student choice in experiential learning. The issue was tackled from a number of points of view:

> Obviously people make a personal choice about how much to divulge of their experience ... I think it is really important to actually give them an opportunity, give them some space and permission to share the effects that the experiential learning has had on them.

Here, the issue is that students should be given the opportunity to talk about what happens to them in an experiential learning encounter, although the decision about what they disclose should be left to the individual student.

A number of respondents were explicit that no student should be coerced into taking part in experiential learning sessions:

> The facilitator will have a responsibility to let them know that they don't have to [take part]. The students need to have that confidence to be able to decide. But if they weren't told in the first place, they wouldn't want to come out with it first and say 'Really, I don't want to do this' because their notion of teaching–learning relationships was still that kind that they had at college.

One respondent noted that offering this voluntariness may take courage on the part of the inexperienced tutor:

> Funny, I have been waiting to see, or expecting, most of the individuals in a group to say 'I'd rather not do that' and then it would be impossible to do the exercise. But it hasn't happened yet. And yet it would be my fear and that could be a danger to the facilitator who is not very comfortable yet in using experiential methods. He may not actually tell learners that they have the right [not to participate] because of the fear that most would abstain from participating.

The fear of students not taking part in experiential learning activities seemed to prove groundless for that respondent. His own experience was that people did take part when offered the opportunity not to do so. Another respondent found this aspect of choice an important one and one that had implications for other aspects of the students' lives:

> It can be very liberating, in the sense of people being made more aware of the options in their lives. They can possibly make choices more systematically, once they see that they can make choices.

The fact of being offered a choice at all, seems to be an important one for that respondent and the suggestion is that one such choice can lead on to others, although why such choices should become more 'systematic' is not clear. Traditional learning methods in nurse training have not normally included an 'opting out' clause or voluntary clause. More usually, students are expected to take part in lessons and lectures and the argument is sometimes used that students should take part in learning encounters because (a) they are undertaking a formal training and (b) they are being paid for their attendance. This is in contrast to colleges of higher education and universities where the accent on compulsory attendance and partici-pation is not the tradition.

The issue for the respondents, here, is not just whether or not students should attend experiential learning sessions but that, given the personal nature of experiential learning, students should not be forced to disclose their thoughts and feelings to others and should be able to reserve the right to decide when and if such disclosure takes place. One respondent appears to be suggesting a gradual approach to such disclosure:

> You could have them do it privately, to begin with – write it down – and they would share it with somebody else in the group. You could, as it were, extend the concept of experiential learning into that process of de-briefing and evalu-ation. Then there could be group discussion if you want to.

Therapy and experiential learning

One respondent expressed concern over whether experiential learning sessions could become psychotherapy sessions. This is a point that devel-ops directly out of the issue of self-disclosure, for self-disclosure is neces-sarily an important element of almost all of the psychotherapies (Shaffer, 1978). The respondent raised a number of issues on this matter:

> I think when you start turning things into therapeutic situations or where the teacher sets themselves up as a 'guru', as a fount of wisdom ... I think that's taking education too far. Unless everyone is agreed that that is what everyone wants to do and everyone has gone there with that in mind ... The worry is that in most situations in nurse education, people have no choice – even though they may appear to be offered it ...

Emotions and experiential learning

The question of whether or not experiential learning should or should not shade over into therapy is complicated further by the fact that many of the respondents discussed the emotional element of experiential learning. Given the personal nature of some elements of experiential learning and given that students are sometimes encouraged to self-dis-close their personal thoughts and feelings, it is perhaps unsurprising that emotions sometimes come to the surface. The respondents in this study seem to have some ambivalence about the issue of whether it was or was not appropriate for students to express strong emotions in a learning situation:

> It hasn't happened often [crying]. On one occasion it happened and it was quite difficult. One thing that I wanted to do was to stop it spreading ... that we'd all end up tackling this particular problem. There was a danger that we'd all become involved in the drama that was going on in this person's life. I think what I did was to play it down at the time and then saw her afterwards and had a chat about it.

Here, the fear seems to be exactly that the learning session was liable to become a therapy session: 'there was this danger that we'd all become involved in the drama that was going on in this person's life'. Therapeutic groups actively encourage such involvement. Another respondent reported:

> I know one of my colleagues has jumped in and touched raw nerves in certain people and has not been able to handle that ... these sorts of things tend to occur sometimes. But the group themselves have been alienated from that person [the colleague]. So I tend to stick with a safe one because I don't feel at the present time that I am skilled, if that is the word to use, in entering any more deeply ... into the areas that touch on the emotions.

This respondent seems to be noting that his colleague was not particularly popular for stirring up the student's emotion, he notes his own lack of skill in handling these sorts of situations but also seems to be questioning the appropriateness of working in the emotional domain, by his querying whether or not 'skill' is the appropriate word to describe the handling of emotional situations.

Another respondent talked about what he perceived as the dangers of an over-emotional learning environment:

> If a person has a very good relationship with his personal tutor, then he can just come back and see them whenever he wants but if you haven't got that relationship, then they might tend to go off with all their feelings ploughed up about something and not feel there is anyone to talk to afterwards.

Another hinted at emotional aspects of experiential learning but seemed to move away from the area thus:

> That is not to say that there isn't an emotional element in them. It is just that there hasn't been any over-emotional outcome.

What is difficult to judge, here, is who is defining the issue of 'over-emotional'. As it is a teacher speaking, then presumably, it is that teacher who is deciding that an outcome is or is not 'over-emotional'. What remains hidden is how the students perceive the issue of the emotions in experiential learning. This question of the difficulty of judging levels of emotional arousal was addressed by another respondent who said:

> It is difficult to judge, of course, whether or not an issue is threatening. For example, if you just ask 'What makes you feel bad?' or 'What have you felt sad about recently?', there is always the danger that you may get into something that is very unpleasant.

Another also illustrated the 'unknown' potential for emotional distress in experiential learning:

> This group of general learners had been given all sorts of specific observational tasks to do but in fact they all ended up crying and it all got quite difficult.

The issue of emotional release in experiential learning sessions seemed, overall, to be focused on two things:

- whether emotional release was appropriate in a learning environment and should or should not be encouraged,
- whether a nurse teacher had the necessary skills to handle emotional release if and when it occurred.

Self-awareness

As we have seen in the first chapter of this book, the notion of 'self-awareness' is very much bound up with that of experiential learning. The first extract in this section illustrates a dialogue between the researcher and a respondent on the issue of what self-awareness is. The respondent, prior to this excerpt, has suggested that experiential learning methods were useful for enhancing student's self-awareness:

> *Researcher:* So what is self-awareness?
>
> *Respondent:* Awareness of one's own needs, one's own wants, one's own fantasies. Awareness of what affects other people, awareness of others as well is tied up with it. What other people's needs and wants are and so on. I keep talking about wants and needs and I am thinking now that they are both feelings – there is a feeling side to that. And feedback, I suppose, are the main things, and being in contact with reality and not being in a world of your own ...
>
> *Researcher:* What does that mean?
>
> *Respondent:* What? Reality?
>
> *Researcher:* Staying in contact with reality.
>
> *Respondent:* With me, it means being in touch with the effect of oneself on others and observing in others how you affect them. And seeing whether there is any correlation between that and between the individuals. I think somebody who is totally unaware of how they affect others is a little bit out of contact with reality and to some extent isolated and alone and possibly in need of help.

This respondent is able to articulate a view of self-awareness as being one that involves awareness of one's own view of one's self and also an appreciation of how others see one. He was also suggesting that the 'person who is in touch with reality' is also a person who takes account of other people's needs and wants. This altruistic view is echoed by another respondent, who used the expression 'personal development' to describe part of what he was trying to achieve through the use of experiential learning methods:

> *Researcher:* So what is personal development?
>
> *Respondent:* Personal development, the way I see it, is the process whereby an individual grows in self-awareness and ability to relate empathically to others. I am pretty concerned about the definitions of empathy. I don't see empathy as being total. I see it as being a balance of being able to be with another person and yet to be quite separate, with the recognition that you can never fully understand another person ... Some definitions of empathy seem to me to be almost a compulsive helping. 'I have got to be with the other all the time'. That would seem to deny the reality of being with oneself, self-concern, self-awareness, assertiveness. I seem to be going round in circles here ...

This respondent seemed to be struggling with concepts of self-development/self-awareness and the need to demonstrate empathy. On the other hand, he is acknowledging what he claims to be the impossibility of complete empathy.

Another respondent took much more of an individualistic approach to the question of experiential learning and self-awareness. He suggested that in considering the experiential learning approach:

> I recommended it not so much for the skills but for what it has done for me. It has actually integrated and synthesized a lot of loose ends, put me more in touch with my weaknesses and how I can go forward in my own life ... which is not an easy thing to do when I want to do my own thing but at the same time I want to accommodate you. It is quite difficult.

Rationale for using experiential learning approaches

In this section, respondents identify general explanations of why they use an experiential learning approach. First, a fairly broad and general explanation:

> [I use them] partly because they were done here, before I came, by the other staff. And partly because I can remember learning things when I was training to be a nurse because we did them and had fun while we were mucking about, making beds with people. But also because they are something I've never forgotten, therefore I think that's why they are a good learning exercise.

This respondent appeared to be reflecting on his rationale as he developed it. He works from a position of 'because they were used before ...', to the fact that they are fun, through to his remembering things from his own past that he never forgot.

Another respondent developed the rationale of using experiential learning methods because he enjoyed using them. He suggested that he used them because:

> I enjoy it. I think that is my main reason, although I am well aware that you can't just do things because you enjoy it. It must be beneficial as well. But I ... have got the very naive belief that if I am enjoying the way I am teaching, I am much more likely to be effective. I think there is a point at which that isn't true, like if I am leaving people behind, or if I am just doing things or saying things because I find them interesting or amusing ...

The respondent seems to take a less 'naive' view than he would let us suppose. Indeed, for him to acknowledge that he is 'naive' in this way is to raise a certain irony: if he were naive, presumably he would be unaware of it, by definition of the term. What he goes on to suggest is that he cannot simply use experiential approaches just because he enjoys them, but also that he accepts responsibility for ensuring that his students 'stay with him'. Another respondent echoed this 'fun' element:

> I feel happy with them. I feel confident in using them. I find them fun and I find them very useful to learn and as far as I am concerned, learning is fun.

Another respondent noted that his rationale for using experiential approaches changed as he became more experienced:

> I used to use them for the sake of using them – 'try this because it is something new' – but I must admit that in the last year or two I don't use them so often now. I tend to try and work things on a workshop basis ... a thematic thing and if there is room for an activity ... I look for ways of presenting parts of it experientially.

This respondent, during the course of the interview, described how he had changed from a 'total' experiential learning approach to one that incorporated elements of both more traditional and experiential approaches. Another respondent acknowledged that he used experiential learning approaches but:

> not a lot. If I am teaching science subjects, perhaps anatomy and physiology, its difficult to role play that ... but then I would use things like setting syndicate work for them, where they actually have a certain set task ... whether you would call that experiential learning, I don't know.

Here, having said that he didn't use experiential learning approaches very much, the respondent went on to ponder as to whether other learning methods could be described as 'experiential learning' – again pointing up the difficulty of defining experiential learning. The question of how much teaching and learning is experiential was developed by another respondent:

> *Interviewer:* Would you say, then, that experiential learning methods can be used right across the board for all topics, for some topics or for very few topics? How would you place them on that sort of continuum?
> *Respondent:* About 50%, I would think ... it would need a bit of ingenuity on the part of the lecturers and facilitators to do any more than that. Some subjects just don't lend themselves to experiential learning.

This leads on to the question of what topics and subjects experiential learning methods were used for by the respondents.

Using experiential learning methods

In the previous section, the debate was more about the question of using experiential learning methods at all. In this section, the focus is more on the ways in which such methods were used. Sometimes, respondents used them for particular topics:

> I think it teaches management techniques.

> I use them for things like counselling – counselling skills.

Some respondents doubted the applicability of experiential learning approaches to certain topics, particularly to the teaching and learning of anatomy and physiology:

I think if you look at pure sessions such as anatomy and physiology, I think you would find it more difficult to drag in always the ideas of the experiential learning concept.

More of the general things like bacteriology, biology, anatomy, physiology, dietetics and straightforward psychology – these are best done by other methods ...

It is interesting to note the first respondent's description of anatomy and physiology as 'pure' and to note the second's expression 'general things like' – it is almost as if both were comparing those topics with other sorts of topics (perhaps with the 'softer' topics of interpersonal skills and communication studies), but this must remain speculation as no further explanation was offered or sought. Meanwhile, another respondent took a very different view:

I think experiential learning is applicable to every subject. All the topics – even biology – are taught experientially.

This respondent is suggesting that experiential learning is applicable to all subjects and also underlines that it is applicable to biology. It is as if the respondent might be in some doubt that it could be applicable for this topic.

On one occasion, the approach seemed to be used for personal reasons:

At the top of my list I would put experiential learning activity. Experiential learning is probably my prime interest.

Like the previous respondent, this one had no hesitation in recommending the widespread use of experiential learning methods for all topics.

Another respondent took a different approach to the issue of what to use experiential learning methods for. She suggested that, rather than tie them to particular topics, choosing them was dependent upon whether they were appropriate as a learning or teaching strategy:

It's like any sort of teaching or learning, isn't it? You have to decide what you want them to get out of it and then the best way to achieve that end. And if it's experiential learning, you work it out that way.

This respondent's approach not only differs in its implication that you don't have to tie methods to topics in teaching and learning but also implies more control by the teacher.

It will be recalled that much of the literature on experiential learning is concerned with negotiated learning and with allowing students to puzzle things out for themselves (Rogers, 1983; Brookfield, 1986, 1987). This respondent took a more structured approach in suggesting that it was the teacher who decided what the students were to learn and who then decided on the appropriate method. An anxiety about whether or not experiential learning approaches allowed you to maintain control in this way was voiced by another respondent:

When you're teaching students, I suppose you have to be open and trust them to do what you want. You can stop at an appropriate time and draw out the experience or draw out what they should have learned. That's another thing. If they haven't actually achieved what you expect them to, you've got to salvage something from the situation, haven't you?

This issue of the 'teacher in control of the learning environment' was echoed by a number of respondents:

You have to stop them now and then and get them to explain how they feel and you have to wind them down again or debrief them afterwards.

You need to give them a sort of strategy and allow them to feel successful.

You have to let people know where they are going and what's expected of them.

If problems have occurred it's because the session hasn't been properly structured. People haven't known what the boundaries are.

This issue of structuring, boundary maintenance and organizational control by the teacher was clearly an important one for a number of respondents and in some contrast to the tendency, in the literature, towards allowing the students to structure their own learning and learning approach – as seen in Chapter 2.

Students' responses to experiential learning

Predictably, perhaps, not all students responded to the use of experiential learning approaches in the same sorts of ways. One respondent reflected on the range of responses thus:

There are all kinds of reactions. I would say that there are some that are very resistant to that approach and don't want to know. You get the whole range. You get, I would say, the majority are interested in it. If you wanted a percentage on it, I would say perhaps 75% enjoy it and another group, perhaps 15–20% are cool towards it and dubious and wonder whether it is of any value to them.

Others noted a positive response to the use of experiential learning activities:

Well, they have a good time. They have a giggle and a bit of fun.

Some group, if you gave them the choice, they would spend the whole block doing experiential stuff.

Some, however, noted more negative responses and for a variety of reasons. One felt that experiential learning methods did not suit everyone and this was the cause of some students feeling uncomfortable using them. Note, however, the word that this respondent uses to describe the students:

I think the other thing is that acting and experiential learning doesn't suit the audience sometimes ...

Consciously or otherwise, this respondent identified a class of students in terms of an 'audience'. This metaphor and the notion of acting is taken into account by another respondent who acknowledge that an air of artificiality was sometimes noted by the students: '"It's not like the real thing", is the classic statement.'

It will be noted in the following section, which identifies the perceptions of the students, that this often was the classic response. Other respondents noted this credibility problem:

> I think some of the other difficulties they have is that they can't see the immediate connection between doing role play and the usefulness of that in their work situation.

> [Some of the problems are] being on display, not understanding the connection . . .

The allusion to acting and the stage was developed by another respondent:

> Some people are just shy, they just don't like getting up in front of six people, let alone 19 others, and play acting . . . They don't like that. They don't like being up on the stage, as it were.

Sometimes, problems associated with the use of experiential learning approaches were put down to the students' familiarity or unfamiliarity with them. If they were used from 'day one' in a course, then they were more likely to be positively responded to by students:

> I was of the opinion that if you started with people from the beginning, that they would be fully receptive to it and they would take it on board and they would be pleased as anything with it. But this is not always true. I think it is the way it is introduced and if you help people to understand the value of it.

> Sometimes they respond with some apprehension, if they haven't used them before. And because of this, we usually start with something that is quite humorous, ice breakers and games with no other purpose than to get them used to experiential methods of learning. And then, when we get on to the more serious things, they become very co-operative: they like it.

> I think what it depends on is how they were first introduced to it.

Sometimes, reactions to experiential learning were seen in terms of the students' previous socialization into learning and teaching methods. This appeared to work both positively and negatively:

> Sometimes you get the 18 year olds who are much happier with it because they have done that type of stuff at college and it is nothing new for them.

> I guess some people, within their previous formalized teaching such as when they are in college or before they come into nursing, are more used to a formalized set-up, where they have notepads and you provide them with diagrams . . .

One respondent linked her own uncertainty with the methods with the reception she got from the students:

Because I wasn't terribly relaxed within myself, I think it was transferred to the learners and they were just as tense as I was. Although they would go through with it, maximum learning didn't take place.

Advantages of the experiential learning approach

One of the most pervasive aspects that was to come out of the interviews with the lecturers in this study was their enthusiasm for experiential learning. Often, they chose the experiential learning approach because either they enjoyed it, or they appreciated the increased involvement it allowed them with students:

The person orientation – I love it. I like being involved, I like the students as people ...

The advantages, the main advantage, that you can guarantee that everybody is active, it is active learning – which you cannot guarantee when you are just standing in front of a class.

I think it can be fun. I think it can be exciting. I think people like doing it. Usually, I find that people love it.

Another advantage that was often cited (and in sharp contrast to what the students had to say on the matter) was that of 'realness'. Many lecturers felt that experiential learning had a 'real' quality that was missing from more traditional methods of teaching and learning:

I think the advantages are that it's as real as you can get. Sometimes it is real. It's actual, real experience. There is no transfer problem with that: it's real. It happened or it is happening.

Yes, it's real. If it's not real, it's as near real as you can get it. Therefore people can try things out, perhaps develop skills and try skills out in a safe situation.

The 'realness' referred to here seems to be in contrast to the lack of realness in more formal learning approaches. Alfred North Whitehead (1932) wrote of 'inert knowledge' and of how lecturers were very good at passing on such inert knowledge. He suggested that, in fact, 'knowledge keeps no better than fish'. The respondents, here, seemed to be suggesting that what made experiential learning real, was the fact that students were bringing to the learning situation their own thoughts, feelings and experiences rather than rote-learning 'dead knowledge'. However, one respondent was not quite so enthusiastic on this point and expressed the view that:

I am sometimes a little sceptical of whether people actually give you the truth when you ask them for their appreciations of their experiences or their understandings of what we have been trying to do.

The respondent is raising an issue that seems to have been neglected in the literature on experiential learning approaches to education. Most of that literature refers to the sharing of experiences by participants, but most tend to take it on trust that people will tell the truth about those experiences. Rogers (1983) seems to take a particularly optimistic view on this issue when he suggests that what needs to happen is for the teacher to trust the students and then they will be more self-disclosing. Jourard (1964) took another optimistic view when he suggested that 'self-disclosure begets self-disclosure'. However, what remains unquestioned is that when people do self-disclose, they will necessarily be honest. Sometimes this perhaps rather naive view percolated through the interviews:

> I am very open with the students. I don't pretend to be able to do any more than they do.

> The advantage as far as I am personally concerned is that you can share things together; yourself with the learners, learners with yourself . . .

> It leaves everybody free, relaxed with each other, more honest with each other.

Whilst the idea of a comfortable atmosphere and a relaxed approach seems likely to promote self-disclosure in group therapy settings, it does not necessarily follow that when people disclose in the fairly public setting of an educational group, they will automatically 'be more honest with each other'. One respondent illustrated a seeming lack of honesty with his students when he reported that:

> It also provides responsibility for one's own learning, so it de-emphasizes the fact that it is the teacher's responsibility for them to learn and without having to say so, I found learners just take it on board, without having to be taught. I have to get whatever is possible out of it and yet you don't have to tell them that.

The respondent seems to be suggesting that the responsibility of the teacher is reduced in experiential learning and yet it is not necessary to openly declare the shift in responsibility and the change of emphasis in learning. It was noted in identifying the disadvantages of the approach that confusion sometimes occurred because students and others were not always sure about lecturers' motives and aims. These disadvantages will now be discussed.

Disadvantages with the experiential learning approach

The lecturers identified a number of disadvantages of the experiential learning approach and these were fairly diverse in nature. Some felt that appropriateness was sometimes a problem:

> Yes, people might abuse it in the sense that they may use inappropriate methods in terms of it is not appropriate for the group they are working with and it doesn't necessarily meet the needs of the group, whilst it may be meeting the needs of the teacher.

This response echoes the problem highlighted in the last paragraph of the last section: it was possible to ask who preferred experiential learning methods the most, the students or the lecturers? Sometimes the appropriateness issue was seen in terms of experiential learning being a bandwagon or a passing fashion:

Some see it is the be-all and end-all in education. It is a panacea in terms of you can teach anything with experiential learning. I am not convinced about that. And some people may abuse it. They may use certain methods or approaches which may be inappropriate to the group.

Everyone is jumping on the bandwagon – a whole concept which is being taken on board and people using what is dangerous stuff sometimes.

The 'dangerous stuff' was sometimes made more explicit:

Some people can't cope with doing anything like role play in front of other people. Some people clearly do have unpleasant experiences. You never quite know what you are tapping into when you set up an experiential exercise ... You never quite know what you are going to unlock.

Learning to use experiential learning methods

We noted above that a number of respondents expressed doubt as to whether they could handle some of the situations that might arise out of using experiential learning methods. This leads to the issue of how lecturers came to be prepared to use such methods in nurse education. Often, the training was minimal or they learned by using the approach themselves:

I don't know if you can actually train. I find that most of what I use now, I learned from other lecturers and working with them and seeing how they do it and how they cope with it and trying it myself.

... the role has no formal training as such.

Just by trial and error, unfortunately. I say unfortunately because we have all experienced negative and positive things. It can have disastrous results, although it depends on what topic you choose and whether you think you are skilled or not. You are your own monitor as far as that is concerned.

For these respondents, the whole issue of training was a rather 'hit and miss' affair, although it could be said that they learned to use experiential learning methods experientially – by direct, personal experience. Not many of those who learned in this way felt themselves to be adequately prepared, which raises a nice paradox about the notion of learning from personal experience. One the one hand, it seemed to be an important value that students were encouraged to learn from direct experience, often in an informal, unstructured environment. On the other, many of the lecturers felt that formal training in experiential learning methods would have helped them.

I would have loved to have gone on an experiential learning methods course, which I think would have been very much to my advantage.

Sometimes respondents had come across experiential learning methods during their tutor's courses at teacher training colleges, although the amount of time allocated to experiential learning on these courses seemed to be variable, as did the outcome and the reception:

While I was at [name of college], I spent one full day so-called 'being taught' how to use experiential methods. That was a laugh really, it really was. We knew better methods than what they were trying to impart to us.

I suppose [my training] would add up to something like 120 hours, I suppose. Some of it was new, some of it was old stuff that I knew myself anyway.

When I was on the tutor's course, [name of teacher] used to take us for relationship skills and I got quite involved in that. I didn't particularly enjoy it that much at the time. In some ways I found it a bit difficult and a bit stressful.

Conclusion

In summary, it can be said that although some of the nurse lecturers found experiential learning difficult to define, many of them felt that it was an active and personal form of learning. They felt that it involved emotional responses and encouraged self-awareness. Generally it was viewed as an enjoyable form of learning but it could sometimes be unreal and embarrassing. Finally, it usually involved facilitation rather than teaching.

The students' perceptions

Next, we review the students' perceptions, by the same method: verbatim quotes and commentary.

Definitions of experiential learning

Some students seemed to echo what they thought their lecturers thought experiential learning was but then were able to make their own modifications of those definitions:

> Well, here in the college, the way the lecturers seem to see it is – say you had a session and it would be like practical things – sort of trying – through the experience you got – trying to make you learn something relevant to whatever, but I suppose in the broader sense, like, you know, working on the wards and things like that.

> [I think of it as] the practical experience we have in college, and what I learn on the wards, and talking to the qualified staff about it. Discussing it with them.

The notion of experiential learning as something more than 'just being taught' was identified by other respondents. Also (and this militates against the suggestion made above, that the students were 'primed' in some way), nearly all of the students had very different perceptions of experiential learning when compared to the lecturers. What makes this important is that it will be recalled that the students were drawn from colleges of nursing in which those lecturers worked. Other definitions of the 'more than teaching' sort, were as follows:

> It means learning which differs from sort of conventional classroom instruction, in that it is something which you use when you use your own experience and you learn from what you've done in the past or you actually learn by going through a practical procedure or some exercise. So it is learning which is centred more around yourself and your life than sort of text book stuff.

> Well it's different from the old style of teaching, rather than the emphasis being on the individual to develop the way they should develop or the way they want to develop, the emphasis in traditional teaching is on a person standing in front of them and giving their views.

By far the most common form of definition, however, was the type that identified experiential learning in terms of learning in the clinical setting, or sometimes as a combination of 'college' learning and 'clinical' learning:

> ... the practical exercises we have in college, and I always think of it as what I learn on the wards and talking to the qualified staff about it. Discussing it with them.

> Well, simply learning by experience. I would have thought of it as over in the college doing role play and I would imagine it would be on the wards left to your own devices as far as the lecturers are concerned.

In the above two extracts, we see the hint of two issues that became important ones in the study: (a) the student's view of the clinical situation and the clinical staff and (b) the student's view of the tutorial staff in the college or college of nursing. The clinical emphasis was to be found in other respondents' responses:

> Experiential learning involves a wide environment of skill, particularly on the wards.

> Well, practically anything that's actually practical and involves doing things is experiential learning, in my opinion – any type of nursing that I've actually done or come across on the ward has been experiential learning to me. What I don't regard it as is learning from books and things – anything theoretical, I don't classify that as experiential learning.

Notable in the last extract is the differentiation between learning on the ward and 'theoretical' learning. Experiential learning, for this respondent, was associated with 'practical' things.

On the other hand, sometimes a more individualistic approach was taken to defining the field: personal learning and the process of learning from life experience, as suggested by some of the nurse lecturers.

> Well, I think experiential learning includes absolutely everything. I think you could argue that your entire life is a learning experience, you could classify anything as experiential learning. Were you thinking of something specific?

This respondent's question of the researcher is interesting as it suggests that the game of 'guess what's in my head' was going on between respondent and researcher (Holt, 1964). Holt argues that it can be frequently noticed that students try to anticipate the 'right answer' for the teacher by 'reading the signs' or checking for clues as to what that teacher might want as an answer. In this interview, it seemed possible that the respondent was trying to please the researcher by coming up with the 'correct' answer.

The individualistic, 'personal' approach to experiential learning was taken by another respondent who suggested that:

> I suppose my views of experiential learning are actually trial and error, by yourself with nobody else telling me what or what not to do.

The themes of learning from personal experience – particularly in the clinical settings – were developed further by all the respondents and it is to that issue that the discussion now turns.

Learning in the clinical setting

It quickly became clear that the students felt that they learned most about nursing from working in the clinical setting. This was often of more importance to them than were the activities carried out in the college of nursing. One student summed this up most completely when she suggested that:

> Well, I suppose that's the job you have got to do and obviously the people on the ward are actually doing it. And you are sort of there, aren't you?

This student invokes a rather passive view of the learning process. For her, it seemed, the process of 'being there' was enough in itself. Others developed this theme:

> I mean, on the wards you learn by ... you don't learn so much by being taught over here [in the college of nursing], you learn when you actually go and do it on the ward.

> Yeah, I definitely learn on the wards. I mean there are sort of theories of psychology and sociology and there are sort of things you can do in the college but I mean, there's everything you can learn on the ward.

Sometimes, this concept of learning on the wards was compared not with learning in the college, but with learning from books. It will be noted in the next section, that the student's view of the college of nursing was not always complementary. In the following extracts, however, the comparisons are between learning from books and learning in the clinical setting:

> Well, it's all right reading it from a book but actually seeing it on the ward – and actually seeing ... like reading about schizophrenia, it is sometimes very difficult to understand unless you actually see a patient displaying thought disorder – like 'thought blocking' – then you can understand it much easier, I think.

> Like with medicine. If you did it just by reading books you probably wouldn't remember the tablets and all the different names. When you are on the ward,

with a qualified member of staff, you remember them because you can see them in front of you – you can see all the different names on them, not just in a book.

Both these students were demonstrating the 'learning by doing' principle, often encountered in the literature on experiential learning and described by the nurse lecturers. However, another notable feature was that they talked about learning by 'seeing'. It would appear that by seeing certain elements of nursing, they feel that they are more likely to remember them. This issue is extended to 'seeing staff' in the next extract.

> To me, learning by seeing people, to me that's the best way. Actually to see something being applied, practically and then I can develop that. I don't tend to pick things up reading from books but if I go and see someone being nursed or you read through care plans or you watch how ... what I tend to do is model from senior nurses if I think they are a good model.

The student, above, demonstrates all of Kolb's stages of the experiential learning cycle but in the clinical setting. First, she describes how she has an experience ('seeing something being applied'). The she reflects on what has happened and applies it to another situation ('and then I can develop that'). She also demonstrates that she makes an assessment of the nursing staff that she sees around her and selects one or more out as a 'role model'. Presumably, though, she has internalized some criteria for what a 'good model' is and it is interesting to raise the question as to where she came upon such criteria. She admits that she does not 'pick things up reading books'; she also acknowledges that learning about nursing, for her is best carried out in the clinical setting. Two possibilities seem likely here: (a) she has reflected on good practice, herself, and decided upon her own criteria for what makes a good role model, or (b) she has internalized teaching about good nursing from the college of nursing but does not make this link explicit.

Sometimes the question of learning in college was explicitly challenged:

> Me, personally, I probably wouldn't remember as much if I was learning in the college, if I was in the college all the time because after so long things tend to go in one ear and out the other, whereas if you are on the wards you remember it.

Another student expressed his feelings about the college of nursing more explicitly:

> Actually, I learn most on the wards. I don't really like being in college much. Yes, on the wards.

Although 'liking being in college' may not be a necessary condition for learning, this response may be compared to some of the nurse lecturers who stressed that the experiential approach to learning was an enjoyable one. It seems, for this student, at least, this was not the case. For one student, too, learning in the college was not so 'real' and no substitute for being in the 'real' situation, i.e. the clinical situation:

> I think learning on the ward, that's the best place you do actually learn. I can remember ... we had one of the sisters come over to the college to teach us and

we had to actually practise on oranges, which is – when we go out on the wards and actually do it on humans – it's nothing like it. I don't think that even when you practise on an orange, you still haven't learned the technique until you actually do it. I think that goes for an awful lot of things. If you get taught from set to set, from week to week, if you have someone demonstrating to you, well, it isn't actually the same as doing it yourself.

Whilst a number of the lecturers felt that they were encouraging the students to practise in a safe setting, it seems that the students often didn't feel that such practice approximated to the 'real thing'. Permeating all of the student interviews was the theme that the 'real thing' was synonymous with 'being in the clinical setting'.

In the final example in this section, the respondent notes not only the importance of learning in the clinical setting but also a perceived transience of the college learning programme:

Well, as I'm on the wards, I have the experience of actually doing the job. You know, when we qualify, or if we qualify, we're not going to be coming back to college ever again, except for things, maybe, like courses. So that what we are really aiming at is for jobs on the wards.

In summary of this section, the feelings and perceptions that permeated most of the students' interviews, with respect to the clinical setting and the college of nursing, were:

- that when it came to learning about nursing, most of that learning occurred in the clinical setting;
- that the college of nursing was not necessarily an important aspect of their learning process.

Experiential learning in the college of nursing

What, then, were the students' perceptions of the sort of experiential learning that took place in the school or college? Sometimes, the students' views were very positive and they would have liked more experiential learning in the school or college:

Respondent: I think it should be a vital part of nurse training and in my view I think that nearly all of our learning should be experiential and I don't think we have enough of it.
Researcher: Which sort are we talking about now …?
Respondent: We're talking about, I think, in the College we should be doing more – more constructive role play. But I find that it's not so much. I don't think in the last two years we've ever had a tutor actually recommend or suggest role play.

Yeah, well, it's quite popular at the moment. Quite the in thing, I suppose. And also because it can work. I think that with certain people, it can work. People can get a lot out of it.

The first respondent above felt that nurse lecturers should use or recommend role play more often. A clue to why they might not is contained in the next section of this analysis, when students' views of role play are discussed. Not all students enjoyed role play. The second respondent, above, noted the present popularity of experiential learning methods, rather dryly, but also acknowledged their value for 'certain people', suggesting, perhaps, that experiential learning methods did not suit every student.

On the other hand, some students were unequivocal in their appreciation of the value of experiential learning methods as an approach to 'doing' rather than just 'listening': 'They're more important that just sitting down and being told. Its much easier to drum it into you I think if you really experience it.'

Another student discriminated between the relative values of certain types of experiential learning activities used in the college:

> Some of the counselling techniques that we sort of role played – I can see them going into practice in the ward and I find that they are helpful when I'm on the wards. The icebreakers and things that we do in a group, we tend to do for our pleasure and enjoyment and I don't think we really use them when we're at work.

What is interesting here is that a number of lecturers commented on the fact that experiential learning activities could be light-hearted and fun to take part in and that they could 'make learning enjoyable'. This respondent is suggesting that the things that she takes part in that are for her 'pleasure and enjoyment' are not things that transfer back to the clinical setting. This, lighter side of experiential learning was commented on by another respondent, thus:

> I think maybe the disadvantage is when you take it as like a comedy at the time. You don't take the serious side of it: you just laugh and joke. You don't think about it seriously and obviously, you're meant to.

This respondent seems clear about the intention of the tutor or about the aim of the activities but acknowledges that he or his colleagues can easily find those activities the subject of mirth. It seems, also, that he is suggesting that because of the laughter, the activity is less than useful.

Linked to the notion of not taking experiential learning activities seriously was another, perhaps more serious theme: the students' view of the college and the lecturers in general. Various negative comments were made about the way in which learning sessions were conducted:

> I wouldn't describe this Nursing College as doing much role play. They usually depend upon the group. They say 'Do you want to do role play?' and if the group say no, then they don't do it.

This appears to be a reference to the ideas suggested by some of the lecturers as 'negotiating' aspects of the learning process. For this student, however, the negotiation process seems to have broken down and the student's tone (from replaying the interview tape) is one of derogation.

Sometimes, experiential learning and a student-centred approach were seen as 'easy options' by the students:

Well, sometimes it's easy for them, sitting down with us. They set you a scene and let you get on with it and they sit back and watch, then tell you what you've done wrong.

A variant on this response was the one offered by this student who felt that the approach to learning lacked structure and clarity:

Sometimes it's a bit wishy-washy because we're not getting any input at all. You have to do it all yourself. So sometimes you get to a point where you don't really know where you're going ...

Again, it is interesting to compare such responses with those of the lecturers, who claimed that they were breaking down barriers between themselves and the students by being more informal and less structured. It would seem that this was not necessarily the 'received' perception. Other respondents were more scathing in their comments about the college and the lecturers, although the first of the next group of respondents is reflective about what the lecturers were trying to do.

Well, I suppose it's very hard for them to think of things for us to do, you know, or people to invent things, you know. I think it's quite sort of a clever idea, really. Well, examples of what we have done, say: you sort of tie your legs together or something or you are blindfolded and someone else has got to lead you around ...

Others, though, were less supportive:

I don't really learn that much in college. The wards, you remember it because you've got an incident you can put into memory. You don't have to remember which book you were reading and because you are doing it all the time, it becomes easier, doesn't it, as you do more.

I don't think we get enough input in the college. We are in for one week every three months but sometimes they haven't got the time to teach us.

In the second of the above extracts, it is difficult to know why the lecturers hadn't got time to teach and the point was not developed by the researcher during the interview.

Sometimes, the complaints about the college and the lecturers revolved around the familiar theme of the tutor's being out of date and out of touch with what was happening in the clinical situation:

To be honest, I feel that everything we've done in the college seems to be a bit irrelevant and sometimes very out dated and I don't feel prepared at all for when I go to a new environment.

It just that sometimes, it is difficult for them to appreciate this – like the common complaint is that they always forget what it's like on the ward once they are in the college. Its difficult for them to appreciate that you haven't just your [college] work: you are working 38 hours a week on the wards.

Like the staff on the wards say, the lecturers should do more, which I think they should come over to the wards more. They don't seem to become involved on the wards and they expect the staff on the wards to do a lot of teaching and they say 'well, we're not lecturers: they've been trained to teach.'

I find the college quite often – this probably sounds like a criticism – but it's like they tend not to be living in the real world. OK, all the lecturers have worked on the wards before and they are all obviously aware of the situation but, yeah, they set examples in text books and the examples we are given in college have nowhere near the complexity of the person you are dealing with on the ward – just don't even come close.

The last student, above, is not only suggesting that the lecturers may be out of date. He is also doing two other things: (a) acknowledging those lecturers' prior clinical experience (even though that might be out of date) and (b) suggesting that the 'examples' that lecturers use are an over-simplification of real life. This may be an important criticism of some of the experiential learning activities in that they always take place away from the 'real' situation and, therefore, can never exactly match the sort of contingencies that can arise in real life.

In closing this section about students' perceptions of the college and the lecturers, one student, in expressing her dissatisfaction with the experiential learning activities that took place in the college, also recommended her own prescription for how things might be. It appears to be very much in line with the theories of experiential learning that advocate learning by direct personal experience:

I feel they are very limited in that whenever you are in college it's very difficult to get away from the fact that you are in an artificial environment, you are always aware that it's a game, if you like. They only give you a limited insight whenever you do role play. I would be tempted to say that if I was in charge of education, I would actually sort of send people off to another health authority, have them admitted in to a ward and then actually get the real feel of what it's like to come in, because unless you've gone through something yourself, you can't actually have that level of empathy with someone.

This may represent the closest suggestion that any student made about learning through personal experience. The idea of 'admitting' students was used as a training device in one college of nursing. In that college, students were asked to spend 24 hours in a wheelchair in order to experience, as nearly as possible, what it felt like to be profoundly handicapped. Clearly, though, the economics of 'admitting' every student to another hospital is unlikely to make the suggestion a particularly practical one.

Just as some of the lecturers were worried about whether or not students would feel 'safe' taking part in experiential learning activities, a number of students expressed their anxieties in this area. Some admitted to feeling considerably less than emotionally safe and the lack of safety often surrounded the issue of self-disclosure. Talking of a particular learning session in a college of nursing, one student suggested that:

I think that they felt as if they had exposed something that they didn't want to expose: they had been exposed to the group . . . I just think it's wrong for people to be so distressed if they don't want to be, in front of everyone else.

Others also talked about the painful process of either 'breaking down' or of self-disclosure:

> Well, I think people can be upset, breaking down in front of everybody ... it shouldn't get to that stage.

Sometimes this discomfort was linked to the issue of voluntariness or the freedom to elect not to take part in an experiential learning activity:

> I think, sometimes if you go into a session and you don't know what you are doing, it can be quite threatening. If somebody explains to you what you are going to do beforehand, and also the fact that if we don't want to do it, we don't have to – I mean, we can just sit and observe.

> Well, we're all sitting round in a group and we were not told what we're doing and we're not given the option to opt out if we want and you don't know what's going to happen. I don't like that.

Role play

The student group could be divided into those who liked role play and those who did not: there were few 'in betweens'. The largest group was those who did not like it.

First, the students who liked it and found it useful. Sometimes, there was a straightforward acknowledgement of it as a learning technique:

> Well, I like role play. I don't think there is a limit to the practical things you can do with it.

> I enjoy it. I enjoy it very much.

> Well, it does sort of reproduce a sort of situation that could happen on the ward. It does make you think of how to put things into practice. What we have learned, sort of like communication skills, body space, posture: so it does sort of help in that it is a less severe atmosphere than on the ward.

> I think role plays were good actually. This was sort of very embarrassing to do, but once you get used to it, I think it's one of the most important exercises that we do.

All of these students were able to make a link between doing the role play and that role play's value as an educational experience. The third respondent above makes explicit reference to how certain interpersonal skills, learnt in the college of nursing, could be carried over into the clinical setting via such role play.

Sometimes, though, there was a 'but' acknowledged in the student's response. Often, this took the form of 'I like it but I know students who don't'.

> I enjoy role play but some people just don't like doing it because they have to put themselves in role positions, they have to see another point of view. They might be quite an immature type of person.

> In my group, they shy away from it, role play exercises, saying it's silly, things like that. There's only really two of us in the group who do enjoy it and get a lot

out of doing role play because we actually try to put ourselves in that position: whereas the others don't really get themselves into that position so I don't think they benefit from it much.

In the first of these cases there is a judgement that people who don't like role play may be immature. In both of the quotations, there is a suggestion that what other people find difficult about role play is the 'putting yourself in someone else's position'. This empathizing aspect of role play was noted by another student who liked role play:

I enjoy role play, but I have found in our set and with a lot of other sets I see doing it, there are people very reluctant to do it. I enjoy it. I feel I learn a lot from it because, you know, role play – you can put yourself in that person's position and see what it was like for them, from their point of view.

The question of learning about empathy and other interpersonal skills, such as counselling was discussed by another student in a largely positive light:

It's artificial in a way, but if you are talking particularly about counselling situations, it is one way of learning to deal with people or talk to people. Role play exercises are good in that way, but then again, it's artificial in a way that it's a story – it's not real – but it's a way of picking up techniques, counselling techniques.

Despite the acknowledgement of the 'artificiality' of the role play situation, the student found role play a useful way to learn counselling methods.

Another student felt that the idea of role play was a good one but that it was not sufficiently or appropriately used. She suggested how it might be made more appropriate to clinical nursing:

Maybe it would be a good idea whereby you do the role play here [in the college] and you do a little bit of it then you're expected to carry it on to the patients, without supervision, but will, like, be sitting in a room where the tutor will be. Then, maybe, it would be the right atmosphere then, when the lecturers come over on the ward. I think one day a week or something, so that the students on the ward could have a role play session. But we should do it there [in the clinical setting] because it's nothing to do with the college.

This student seemed to be acknowledging a variety of things. First, she seemed to feel that role play could be useful (in that she was suggesting its use at all). More than that, however, she was seeing it as a possible way of integrating the tutorial staff from the college of nursing into the clinical setting. It is almost as though she was offering it as an 'excuse' for the lecturers to visit the wards – that it offered them a definite role in the clinical setting. She noted, too, that role play had 'nothing to do with the college'.

Returning to the issue of why some people did not like role play, we return to the issues of being able to 'act', to take on the role of another person. A number of students felt that the 'acting' aspect of the role play made them either embarrassed or made them doubt the value of the role play on the grounds that it was 'artificial'. One student appreciated the artificial aspect and saw it as a positive and educational factor:

> When I do role play in the classroom, everybody's aware that it's a false situation and maybe an ideal situation, so it's good, in a way, to feel that you can make mistakes in the classroom and it doesn't really matter.

Others, though, were less certain of the value of it and found that the embarrassment and unreality factors seemed to get in the way. Often, too, they supported the idea that role play appealed to certain sorts of people: often more extrovert people than themselves.

> Well, people who don't mind performing in front of a group like it. I would say, generally, that more extrovert people like it.

> Well, role play is embarrassing: standing up in front of everyone else, you know, and having to do something. Whereas if you sit and do something slightly more practical, if everybody's doing it, then the spotlight isn't on you.

> I think it's too much of a false situation. I try to sit and watch with other people and learn a bit from it but I don't do it myself. I'll do other things, but not specifically role play.

> I think role play is OK if you feel comfortable doing it but personally I fell silly doing it so I don't do it now.

The last two respondents, in suggesting that they 'don't do it' imply that they have choice in whether or not they take part. Also, the first of those two suggests that she learns vicariously, by watching others doing role play. The second respondent, above, seems to be highlighting the need not to be 'put on the spot' but to be allowed to feel part of the group. The issues of choice and of different teaching and learning methods suiting different people was taken up by another student:

> I just know that some people say 'I don't like role play, I'd rather not do it.' And since it's generally a voluntary thing you are not held to do this or that or the other. Maybe it's because they don't think that role play is of any value in learning. Some people very much like the conventional teaching approach and think that the only kind of proper teaching is where they have got somebody sort of telling them a list of facts and then writing it down. Some people are happier with that. I don't think that's a kind of criticism of them. That's just: people have different preferences.

Here, then, role play was being compared to more 'traditional' learning and teaching methods: an allusion made by a number of the nurse lecturers. The respondent also suggested that various methods may suit different people, even though his comments about some people thinking that the 'only kind of proper teaching' involves listening and taking notes, seemed to contain a negative evaluation of such people.

Experiential learning methods

It is interesting to note the sorts of experiential learning methods that students said they had taken part in. A wide range of exercises and activities were identified by the students and that range covered most of the activities described in the literature as 'experiential learning methods' and those described by the lecturers.

> We have had role play, small group exercises, empathy exercises, ice-breakers, games, those sorts of things.

> We have done other things like being blindfolded and tied up and so forth and we've done role play and psychodrama.

> We've done psychodrama and lots of exercises.

These quotations represent what many of the students repeated: that they had taken part in a wide range of activities that could be called 'experiential learning activities'.

Advantages of experiential learning

A number of the students made links between the various approaches to experiential learning in the college of nursing and the value of those approaches in terms of the clinical setting.

> For me, it [experiential learning] linked up in a way that I can develop counselling techniques. Although artificially, I can develop techniques, judge situations, body language, posture, tone of voice – putting yourself in an artificial situation stimulates response and that is useful and helps me in the ward.

Here the acknowledgement was made that the activities used produced an 'artificial' situation but that situation was both useful and clinically applicable.

On a similar but different note, some students found the use of blindfolds to simulate blindness and activities in which they were encouraged to imagine what it was like to hallucinate, or be handicapped, useful, as it made them reconsider their attitudes and feelings towards blindness, schizophrenia and disablement. They were able to describe their progress through such activities:

> I think as far as the blindfolding was concerned – I think sort of actually telling, actually teaching a class of nursing, telling them what it's like to be blind – I still don't think you can appreciate it, what it's like. I suppose being blindfolded is really putting you in the situation to some extent. It's then that you really appreciate what it's like and really empathize ... It's like the same for schizophrenia and things. You know this person is hearing voices and you've no experience what it's like and you have to counsel that person, perhaps. But actually sitting there with earphones on and having a voice whisper to you just shows that it can be frightening. It modifies your attitude to a great extent, that sort of exercise. I mean, actual formal teaching isn't so likely to modify that.

> The empathy exercises we had I thought were good, actually, because we did exercises where we were actually blindfolded. We had an arm in a sling and you had to be led around for quite a while by another member. Yes, it did make – give you an understanding of what it must be like being blind or handicapped in some way. So I thought those exercises were very good.

Some difference may be noted between the above 'simulations' and role play. In the simulations referred to above, the students were put in a situation, by the use of 'props' to help them to experience sensory or motor deprivation. In role play, however, they were asked to play another person. In the former situation, the students were helped to experience the world from another person's point of view through active intervention on the part of the lecturers. In the role play situation, the students had to imagine what another person's world might be like. Arguably, the more concrete 'simulation' allowed for a more dramatic appreciation of other people's lives. Also, the simulation encouraged the students to undertake stages in Kolb's (1984) experiential learning cycle, discussed in Chapter 1. They were offered an experience (e.g. being blindfolded) and they reflected on that experience and then carried the learning over into the 'real' situation. In one case, above, the student felt that this 'modified your attitude' and noted that the doing of this activity was more likely to produce such attitude change than would more traditional, formal teaching. This issue of 'experiencing' was taken up by another student:

> If you learn about something and you actually experience it, then that's when it sinks it. In the same way if you have a piece of research to do rather than picking up a book and reproducing it verbatim, you actually go out and experience the research yourself. That's the way that you learn and it's more beneficial in that way because you are actually going through the situation.

The 'going through the situation' may be the key to the students' perceptions of learning and remembering. Throughout the interviews students frequently referred to learning in the clinical setting rather than in the college of nursing. Others, as we have noted, thought that 'seeing' a situation made much more sense to them than reading about it or 'being taught' about it. Given that the major part of the life-world of the student is the clinical setting and given the frequent suggestions by them that 'doing' is better that 'being taught' it would seem that experiential learning as perceived by the students has much to do with learning by being personally involved and immersed in the learning situation: being active rather than passive learners. A number of students tried to put this into words:

> Well, I suppose it makes you look at things in a different way, you know. An experience, I suppose. Well, it's not learning as in remembering, it's just – I suppose you remember what you've experienced better. You apply it, perhaps. No, you can apply it because it means more to you, perhaps.

For this student, capturing the essence of what experience meant was not easy but he seemed to be conveying this sense of the primacy of experience itself, rather than having just 'remembered' things. Another student developed this theme in a personalized way. He saw experiential learning as concerned with 'personal knowledge' rather in the way that it was discussed in Chapter 1:

> You'd be involved more as an individual person. Nobody else would have your knowledge, your skills, because it's your view on a particular subject;

it's your view on say, psychology. If you are looking at a particular subject and you read that, then you develop your own views and your own particular perspective.

Another student was able to distinguish between this process of learning from personal experience and another domain of 'factual knowledge':

I think, as with the case of the blindfold, you might know someone who's blind and perhaps your own previous life experience may influence your reaction to it. I think you do need, as well as learning from experience, you do need the sort of factual backup from the college, the theory.

This student seems to be acknowledging the limitations of personal experience and suggesting that theoretical and factual knowledge are important alongside the more personal or experiential knowledge (Heron, 1981).

It is here that we have come full circle. It will be noted in this analysis that students often began by describing experiential learning as learning in the clinical setting, in the 'real world'. Here, in closing, we see that view confirmed and enlarged a little to take account of experiential learning being personal learning, learning by doing and learning by being involved in what is happening, as opposed to 'traditional' textbook, college or 'remembering things' learning. Among the things that distinguish the student's view of experiential learning from the educator's view are that the lecturers tended to elaborate the concept of experiential learning with reference to 'philosophies of teaching and learning' – particularly the humanistic philosophy. The students appeared to take a more pragmatic view: 'I learn things by doing them'. Also, the lecturers tended to emphasize the role of self-awareness and self-disclosure in the learning process, whilst the students were quite often embarrassed by such issues and preferred to choose their own rate of self-disclosure.

Conclusion

In summary, it can be said that the students tended to view experiential learning in clinical and practical terms. They also saw it as a personal and active approach to learning and one that may not be popular if it involves role play. The students also noted a divide between clinical learning on the one hand and 'college' learning on the other.

This chapter has explored something of the diversity of experiential learning through the reporting of a descriptive study of the topic. It will be noted, as always, that the differences between the *prescriptions* contained in books and the *practice* of everyday life are often marked and show through in the study reported in this chapter.

Recommended reading

Drummond, A. (1996) *Research Methods for Therapists*. Cheltenham, Nelson-Thornes.

Morse, J.M. and Field, P.A. (1995) *Nursing Research – The Application of Qualitative Approaches*, 2nd edn. Cheltenham, Nelson-Thornes.

5

Using Experiential Learning Activities

This chapter offers concrete guidance on the use of the exercises for inter-personal skills development offered in the final two chapters. Each exercise is laid out under a series of headings and these are identified below. First, though, a rationale for this type of training.

The gymnasium principle

Exercises of the kind described in this book explore small portions of human behaviour, thought and feelings. On their own, they are likely to be of limited value – although this is not always the case. Mostly, though, they are best used as a *series* of activities, where one leads naturally on from the other. A metaphor that is sometimes used to describe this sequencing is referred to as the *gymnasium principle*. Just as a gymnast tends to exercise discrete sets of muscles – first this set and then that – so the person who is training in interpersonal or human skills can practise a particular aspect of those skills. Then, like the gymnast, after the exercises, the benefits of the 'micro' approach pay off in the 'real world'. Just as the gymnast feels healthier in all sorts of ways after his or her activities, so the nurse who is using interpersonal skills exercises can transfer his or her new skills to the clinical, educational or management setting. On, then, to the headings that are used in the final three chapters of this book.

Aim of the activity

Here, the intention of the activity is made clear. What can never be written for such exercises is a series of behavioural objectives. As we have noted throughout this book, experiential learning is necessarily idiosyncratic. It is not possible to predict the outcome of a particular exercise for any particular person. All that can be said is that there is a clear intention in setting out to offer the exercise as a learning activity. On the other hand, it is important not to be too wide-eyed an innocent about this. Once these activities have been used a number of times by a particular facilitator, he or she will come to recognize certain typical patterns of response. These can help in shaping future courses and in the development of new activities and exercises.

Number of participants recommended

Whilst a minimum and maximum figure is quoted for each activity, many of the activities can be adapted for larger numbers. Many, too, can be carried out by only two persons, learning as a pair. If larger numbers are being catered for, it is important that a great deal of structure is used in organizing the exercise. In groups of 20 and above, it is helpful if the instructions for the activity are written out in the form of a pre-prepared handout, so that everyone is clear about how to proceed. It is also helpful if, during the feedback and processing session, the larger group is broken up into smaller groups of about four or five people. Many do not like discussing their experience in a large group and constraints of time may mean that not everyone gets heard in a larger group. A chairperson may be nominated or elected in each feedback group. A short plenary session with the whole group may be facilitated afterwards as a means of maintaining group cohesion.

Environmental considerations

The usual suggestion, here, is that group members sit round in a circle. Such a circle is symbolic of unity and also ensures that the group facilitator is on an equal footing with the group and not physically (and symbolically) set apart from it. It is important, too, that the group does not sit around a table or in front of desks. In this way, there are no physical barriers between participants. The arrangement also allows for greater ease of movement if the exercise calls for the group's splitting into pairs or smaller groups.

Equipment required

None of the exercises calls for difficult to obtain equipment. The most important feature of the exercises is the personal one: the meeting of people to enhance their skills.

Time required

Taking time over these activities is very important. None of them should be rushed and plenty of time should be allowed for the discussion part of the activity. If the activities take significantly shorter time to complete than is suggested in the text, it is worth reflecting on what parts you are hurrying. The most frequently rushed part of the activities is the *reflective* part, when group members reconvene and discussed what happened. This is a shame, for this period of reflection and discussion is the most important of the whole activity. So ... take your time!

The process

This section, in each case, offers a clear, stage-by-stage account of how to run the exercise. Initially it is useful if these instructions are followed to the letter. Once the facilitator and the group have become familiar with the approach, various modifications can be made to suit the circumstances. Many of the most effective activities are those that the facilitator devises personally. On the other hand, as was noted above, it is important that none of the exercises is rushed.

Evaluation

This section offers questions that the facilitator may want to ask of the group. They are meant as guidelines only. Clearly, the questions that arise out of the process of the group activity are far more useful than any preconceived ones. It is hoped, though, that the questions in these sections stimulate ideas for your own questions.

Notes

Sometimes there are variations on an activity which can be used in different situations to explore different aspects of interpersonal skills. These notes offer suggestions for such variations and, sometimes, lead the way to further reading.

Using the activities

A useful procedure for planning the use of these exercises is outlined in Figure 5.1, an experiential learning plan. Example programmes for teaching counselling skills and for teaching group facilitation skills are also offered at the ends of the next two chapters.

In the cycle in Figure 5.1, a short theory input is offered if the exercise is to be used in a classroom. If it is to be used in a peer learning group, a discussion or reading period may be substituted for this stage. The theory input should be kept fairly short and to the point and should not become a full-blown lecture. The aim of such a theory input is to set the scene and to offer a minimal theoretical framework through which students can test some of their experiences.

Second, the aim of the experiential exercise is introduced to the group. It seems reasonable to tell the students what you have in mind when you ask them to undertake an activity, although there are problems here too. If you are *too* explicit about your aims, you stand to limit the student's own perceptions of what they experience. They will be looking to satisfy your aim. On the other hand, to suggest that you have *no* aim in mind seems naive if not dishonest! No one suggests an activity for no reason at all!

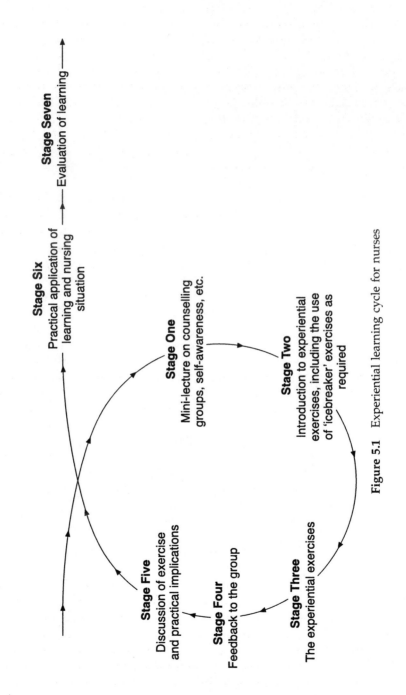

Figure 5.1 Experiential learning cycle for nurses

Stage Seven — Evaluation of learning

Stage Six
Practical application of learning and nursing situation

Stage One
Mini-lecture on counselling groups, self-awareness, etc.

Stage Two
Introduction to experiential exercises, including the use of 'icebreaker' exercises as required

Stage Three
The experiential exercises

Stage Four
Feedback to the group

Stage Five
Discussion of exercise and practical implications

Third, the exercise is carried out as outlined. Following the exercise, all participants feed back their experiences to each other and to the group. Out of this feedback can be developed a fruitful discussion and the learning that has taken place may become the basis for practical use in the 'real' nursing situation.

Finally, the learning is applied and the nurse carries his or her new skills into the clinical area or into the community. This is the crucial test of the experiential learning method: that skills are transferred from the classroom to the clinical setting. *How* this occurs is fraught. One way of encouraging such transfer is for tutors and lecturers to ensure that nurses receive sufficient clinical support and to ensure that they, as teachers of the skills, are seen in the clinical areas as credible role models as well as teachers.

The experiential learning cycle can be evaluated through further discussion at a later date and further repetitions of the learning cycle carried out. The learning cycle, then, combines experiential learning from the clinical setting with experiential learning in the school or college and back again. The stages are now described in more detail.

Stage One

The mini-lecture or theory input should be a short theoretical exposition of the particular topic being explored. The aim, as we have seen, should be to create a theoretical framework through which students can make sense of their coming experience. There is no reason why such a theory input has to be given by the facilitator. It is often better given by a student or by a group of students. A useful method is to split the student group into smaller sub-groups and invite each of the sub-groups to research and give a short input on one aspect of the topic. What is to be avoided at all costs, however, is students' reading lengthy papers on the topic. A short series of headings and one or two main references will often suffice. It is probably better to underteach than to overteach.

Stage Two

A concept of experiential learning is introduced briefly and clearly. Any questions about the nature of the exercises are answered in a straightforward manner and students are offered the option of either taking part or observing their colleagues. One of the aims of this part of the session should be the 'demystifying' of the students. Students have often been socialized into fairly traditional expectations of what teachers and learners do. To suddenly overwhelm them with activity-based learning is not a good plan. Nor is the 'try it and see' approach: students are generally more comfortable if they know a little of what to expect in advance.

Before the exercises are carried out, it is sometimes of value to use one or more 'icebreakers'. These are short activities carried out by the group which serve to create a relaxed and open atmosphere in which group members can enter more fully into the exercise being undertaken. A selection of such exercises are describe here: others may be found in a number of publications listed at the end of this book. Most are light-hearted and should be treated as such. Similar icebreakers or variants of these activities can be found in a variety of sources (see, for example: Heron, 1973; Pfeiffer and Jones, 1974; Kilty, 1982). In a useful book of icebreakers, Jones (1991) has this to say:

> The metaphor of icebreaking is apt. An icebreaker is a vessel designed to clear a passage in frozen waters and open up channels of communication. In human terms icebreakers are intended to deal with frosty situations, cold starts, nervous freezing. They aim not only to break ice but also to warm the atmo-sphere. A 'warm-up' is another name for an icebreaker. By contrast the social mixing and introductions in everyday life are very hit and miss. They can be difficult: one can forget names, not know what to say, and if embarrassment turns into panic then the mind can go completely blank or one can burble like an idiot. An icebreaker helps to overcome such problems.

Opinions about the use and appropriateness of icebreakers vary. Some people like using them and some loathe their use (Hopkinson, 1994). Some students enjoy them and find them helpful, other find them embar-rassing. My own experience is that younger people, for whatever reasons, find them easier and more helpful than do older people. The general rule, here, perhaps, is to try them and see what happens. If the group that you are working with don't like them, start sessions off in another way.

Some facilitators use icebreakers as a form of introductory activity with new groups of students or at the beginning of a workshop. Another format for such introductions is as follows.

The facilitator invites each person, in turn, to identify the following things about themselves:

- their name (or the name they prefer to be known by)
- their current job,
- three things about themselves that are unconnected with work.

Alternatively, the group can be divided into pairs and the members of the pairs interview each other. After about 10 minutes, the pairs return to the group and each person is then introduced to the group by their partner.

Icebreakers

1 Milling and pairing

Group members stand and move and wander around the room. At a signal from the facilitator they stop and pair off with the person nearest to them. The pairs spend a few minutes sharing thoughts on one of the following:

(a)   a recent pleasant experience
(b)   two interests away from work
(c)   feelings about the group or about the workshop.

2   *Mirroring*

Group members wander around the room and periodically stop in front of each other. When they do so, each pair attempts to mirror the body position and facial expression of the other.

3   *Sculpture*

Group members pair off. One member then moves and positions the other, as a shop dummy might be moved. The group members being sculpted in this way stay in the positions into which they have been put. The 'sculptors' then wander around and view each other's work.

4   *A piece of music ... a book ...*

The facilitator asks members in turn to describe themselves in one of the following ways:

(a)   'If you were a piece of music, what would you be? Describe yourself as that.'
(b)   'If you were a book, what book would you be? Describe yourself as that.'
(c)   'If you were a building, what building would you be? Describe yourself as that.'

5   *Compliments*

Group members complete a 'round' in which they turn to the person on their left and complete the sentence: 'What I like most about you is ...'
   Other sentences that can be used here include:

'I imagine that you are ...'
'I would like to be like you for this reason ...'
'I appreciate ...'.

6   *Awareness*

Group members complete a 'round' in which they turn to the person on the left and complete the sentence: 'Now I am aware of ...'. They complete the sentence by noticing something about the person sitting on their left. Group members are encouraged not to rehearse their responses but to respond spontaneously as their turn comes.

7   *Formative experiences*

Group members recall three formative experiences from their lives to date and share those experiences with the group. The experiences should be positive ones.
   Some of these icebreakers will be easier to carry out and take part in than others. Much will depend on how well group members know each other. If a light-hearted, open manner is adopted by the facilitator, many people will find them easy, amusing and sometimes revealing. Others will not and no one should be forced to take part in an icebreaking activity that they are not happy to undertake.

Stage Three

In this stage, the experiential learning exercises described in the following chapters are carried out.

Stage Four

Following the exercise, group members are invited to feed back their experiences of the exercise. Usually a broad open question such as 'What happened?' will be sufficient to encourage people to share what happened during the activity. It is important that each member is allowed to contribute as he or she sees fit and is 'heard'. On the other hand, it is not the facilitator's role to make sure that *everyone* has a say. A participant's choice to say nothing should be respected.

This stage of the cycle should be as lengthy as necessary to ensure that all that needs to be shared *is* shared. It is probably during this reflective phase that most new learning occurs. This is equivalent to part of the 'transformation of knowledge' phase of Kolb's learning cycle, discussed in Chapter 2.

Stage Five

During the fifth stage, new learning from the shared experience is applied in a practical way. Group members discuss the application of what has been learned to the clinical or community nursing situation. Thus, if a counselling exercise has been carried out to develop listening skills, the group considers ways in which the nurses present could use their new listening skills to enhance patient care. Sometimes is can be helpful if psychodrama or role-play is used here, to rehearse the process of using the particular skill. It is useful, too, if group members undertake to try out a new skill the day that it is learned – away from the group. In this way the new learning is reinforced, becomes more real and is better remembered. There is a great danger of experiential learning activities producing skills that are then not transferred to the clinical situation. The experiential learning session becomes an interesting but historic 'island' in group members' memories.

Stage Six

This stage, the stage of practical application, takes place away from the classroom. It is the stage in which theory is transformed into practice and in which the new human skills are practised. It is a time of trial and error but also of discovery. It is a time of testing out 'what worked in the learning session' against 'what happens in the clinical setting'. If the gap between the two is too great, then the temptation will always be to slip back to old patterns of behaviour that worked in the past. Application of new learning takes courage and it is here that students will need plenty of clinical support.

Self-monitoring is essential in this stage and it helps if students are encouraged to keep a journal or diary. A modified version of the journal format, described here, has been used at the School of Nursing Studies, University of Wales College of Medicine, as part of a continuous assessment procedure during the Bachelor of Nursing course, during student's psychiatric nursing secondment. It has met with varying amounts of success. After an initial period of the students' feeling that they would not be able to complete the journal, a number found it particularly useful and planned to continue to use it throughout other parts of their course. Others continued to find it difficult to use and one never completed it.

The instructions for completion of the journal are simple. Participants are required to make weekly entries in a suitable book under the following headings:

- Problems encountered and how they were resolved.
- How new skills were applied.
- New skills required to be learned.
- Personal growth issues/self awareness development.
- Other comments.

These headings can be varied according to the needs and wants of a particular group using the journal approach. No guidelines need to be given regarding the amount that is written under each heading. The finished product need not be an 'academic' piece but should be a free representation of the student's experience.

Group members are encouraged to make regular entries and this regularity tends to make the process of keeping the diary easier. Participants who try to 'catch up' and complete the whole thing in one last go tend to have difficulty in remembering what has happened and generally the process is less valuable.

Stage Seven

This seventh stage is the stage of evaluation of both the experiential learning and of the practical application of that learning. Depending on how you define 'experiential learning', it may be argued that *both* these aspects are examples of experiential learning: there is the learning from the group and the learning from practical experience. The following is a useful format for carrying out such an evaluation.

1. Each group member gives feedback on (a) the negative and (b) the positive aspects of his or her performance. It is important that this order is observed so that individuals end their own self-evaluation on a positive note.
2. The group member who has thus self-evaluated invites comments from the group and the tutor or lecturer, again on the negative and then the positive

aspects of his or her performance. This will only apply if colleagues of the teacher have been actively involved with that person during their time in the clinical setting.

An alternative method, as we have noted above, is to use the diary or journal as the basis of self-evaluation. This can be done in one of two ways:

1. Each person meets with a tutor or lecturer and discusses the diary with the educator. Or
2. The peer group meets and all of the diaries and all of the experiences are discussed in a group setting. Out of this group meeting can emerge the general aims of the next learning session.

These processes incorporate both self- and peer evaluation. Such a combination is valuable in that it encourages both reflection by individuals on their own performance and feedback from others. Luft (1969) argues that both self-disclosure and feedback from others are the two vital ingredients for self awareness.

If self-and peer evaluation are two aspects of feedback to students, then the third element is feedback from the tutor/lecturer or sister/charge nurse. If three reports of a given person are obtained in this way, 'triangulation' has taken place (Figure 5.2). Hopefully, the student receives an important mixture of both subjective and objective evaluation data.

Continuing the cycle

Once a round of the cycle has been complete, the learning gained can be carried forward into a new cycle. Nurse education and training

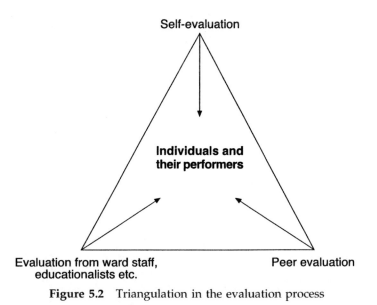

Figure 5.2 Triangulation in the evaluation process

programmes using a module scheme can incorporate the experiential learning cycle into curriculum plans to create a continuous cycle of experience, reflection, learning and application, thus operationalizing experiential learning theory.

The next chapters describe a series of experiential exercises that may be used to develop human skills: (a) in the one-to-one interpersonal relationship (counselling skills) and (b) in the one-to-group relationship (group and facilitation styles). The final chapter offers a number of exercises for the development of self-awareness: awareness that can enhance both counselling and group skills.

Recommended reading

Burnard, P. (1996) *Acquiring Interpersonal Skills – A Handbook of Experiential Learning for Health Professionals*, 2nd edn. Cheltenham, Nelson-Thornes.

6

Experiential Exercises for Human Skills: 1 Counselling Skills

Counselling may be described as a therapeutic conversation between two people in an understanding atmosphere. The breadth of such a definition is intentional and aimed to cover a whole range of situations that may be described as 'counselling'. Consider, for example, the following:

- talking to a person who is about to undergo an operation and who is confused and upset
- discussing progress in the clinical situation with a student nurse
- helping a colleague to reach a decision about a career change
- talking to a person who is worried about HIV/AIDS.

Arguably, all of these situations are situations in which counselling skills are used. The skills that are often associated with professional counsellors are also those that are required by the professional nurse.

In recent years, a range of questions about *what* counselling is, *who* should do it and whether or not it *works* have been asked, both in the literature and in the national newspapers. As consumers become more aware of their rights and more discerning about the nature of the treatments that they are offered, they are – appropriately – asking questions about whether or not counselling is a 'good thing'. The question remains unanswered, convincingly, at the time of writing this book. All we can surmise is that talking about things seems to help a lot of people. Whether or not 'formal counselling' makes a long-term difference has yet to be clarified. In the meantime, a useful distinction, for nurses, can be made between *counselling* and *using counselling skills*. It is argued that the *latter* are of particular use to the nurse.

What, then, are the differences between the two concepts? *Counselling*, it might be argued, is something that is carried out by people whose job it is to counsel. Such people will be known by the job title 'counsellor' and it seems likely that they will pursue this job on a full-time basis. *Counselling skills* are part of the things that they use to pursue that job. Such skills, however, are also transferable to other jobs and, in particular, to nursing. Nurses – without being 'counsellors' in the strict sense of the word – can use a range of counselling skills to help their patients talk through problems, express feelings and make decisions. Such nurses do not practise as counsellors but use the skills that are available appropriately and carefully.

Is counselling effective?

The question often arises as to whether counselling 'works'. A similar but perhaps clearer question is 'is counselling effective?' This section offers a short review of some of the current thinking in this area (at the date of the preparation of this book – August 2001). It is based on a publication by the NHS Centre for Reviews and Dissemination (at the University of York), Vol. 5, Issue 2, August 2001, *Counselling in Primary Care*.

The primary interest of those collating evidence for clinical effectiveness, through systematic reviews of the research literature, is the randomized controlled trial or RCT. The use of RCTs to evaluate counselling and other psychological therapy treatments is contentious (Hazzard, 1995; Seligman, 1995; Roth and Fonagy, 1996; Bower *et al.*, 2000). However, a number of RCTs of counselling in primary care have been conducted.

Rowland *et al.* (2001) published a systematic review of counselling in primary care. The latest update of the review includes seven RCTs of counsellors trained to the standard recommended by the British Association for Counselling and Psychotherapy (Boot *et al.*, 1994; Friedli *et al.*, 1997; Harvey, 1998; Bedi *et al.*, 2000; Bower *et al.*, 2000; Sibbald *et al.*, 2000; Ward *et al.*, 2000; Chilvers *et al.*, 2001). The review focused on counsellors meeting these standards as they are increasingly recognized as a useful benchmark in primary care. The counsellors in these trials treated patients with mild to moderate mental health problems (such as anxiety and depression) referred by GPs. In six of the trials, the comparison group was 'usual GP care' including support from the GP within normal consultations, medication and referral to mental health services.

One RCT used a comparison group of 'GP antidepressant treatment' and was considered separately. The results of six RCTs (with 772 patients) indicated that counselled patients demonstrated a significantly greater reduction in psychological symptoms such as anxiety and depression than patients receiving usual GP care when followed up in the short term (up to 6 months). Psychological symptoms were measured using validated questionnaires such as the Beck Depression Inventory and General Health Questionnaire. These psychological benefits were modest: the average counselled patient was better off than approximately 60% of patients in usual GP care (if counselling and usual care were equally effective, the proportion would be 50%). There were no significant differences between counselling and usual care in the four RCTs (with 475 patients) reporting long-term outcomes (8 to 12 months).

Generally, the RCTs reported high levels of patient satisfaction with counselling (Boot *et al.*, 1994; Hemmings, 1997; Simpson *et al.*, 2000) and that patients were more satisfied with counselling than with usual GP care (Friedli *et al.*, 1997; Sibbald *et al.*, 2000) However, this comparison of GPs and counsellors is difficult to interpret due to the differences in time each has available to spend with patients (Lai *et al.*, 1998).

Two RCTs have compared counselling with other mental health treatments routinely provided in primary care (Ward *et al.*, 2000; Sibbald *et al.*, 2000; Bedi *et al.*, 2000; Chilvers *et al.*, 2000). The first compared counselling with cognitive-behaviour therapy provided by qualified psychologists (Bower *et al.*, 2000; Sibbald *et al.*, 2000; Ward *et al.*, 2000). There were no differences between the two therapies in their overall effectiveness at short- or long-term follow-up. Both therapies were superior to usual GP care in the short term, but provided no significant advantage in the long term.

The second RCT (Bedi *et al.*, 2000; Chilvers *et al.*, 2001) compared counselling with antidepressant treatment provided by GPs who were given specific guidelines on antidepressant use. However, the study was designed to reflect antidepressant prescribing as routinely provided by GPs, and the prescription of medication was not standardized. There were no differences in outcomes between patients receiving counselling and medication at 8 weeks or 12 months follow-up.

Some applications of counselling skills in nursing

Counselling and counselling skills have been widely described in the nursing literature. As a source of references to this literature, this section offers a brief overview of the ways in which writers have reported the use of such skills.

Jones (1990a,b,c) has described how counselling skills can be used effectively in caring for those who are terminally ill. The author demonstrates how empathy, self-awareness and an understanding of mental defence mechanisms can all help in this situation. Lugton (1989), Hopper (1991) and Wyatt (1993) have described how counselling skills have been of value in helping those who are terminally ill and their relatives to come to terms with what is happening. Others have written of counselling in child abuse (Briggs, 1992; Daniel, 1992) and, in particular, how group counselling can be of value in this delicate field. Miller (1991) offers a description of how she used counselling in caring for a man in a special hospital and how basic counselling and negotiating skills can be effective in this specialized environment.

Mok (1989), Bond and Rhodes (1990) and Bond *et al.* (1990) have all written extensively about the use of counselling skills in relation to AIDS counselling. AIDS counselling, it might be argued, is so specialized and so particular that it, understandably, has a literature of its own. Miller and Bor (1992) and Miller, Goldman and Ormanese (1993) are just two examples of the extensive literature in this field.

In another context, Jennings (1992), Lindell and Olsson (1991) and Kwast (1992) describe the role of counselling in settings where the nurse works in a fertility clinic. Cullinan (1991) outlines the value of 'listening visits' for health visitors who visit their clients. It would seem, from this brief review of some of the literature, that counselling and counselling skills have been widely used in a range of nursing settings.

Personal qualities of the nurse as counsellor

Counselling in nursing requires at least two things: (a) the development of certain personal qualities and (b) the learning of basic interpersonal skills. Three clusters of personal qualities identified by humanistic therapist and educator Carl Rogers (1967, 1983) as necessary for an effective therapeutic relationship were:

1. Warmth and genuineness.
2. Empathic understanding.
3. Unconditional positive regard.

The three clusters of qualities are now briefly described and related to nursing.

Warmth and genuineness

Warmth, in the nursing relationship refers to being approachable and open to the patient or colleague. Schulman (1982) argues that the following characteristics are involved in demonstrating the concept of warmth: equal worth, absence of blame, non-defensiveness and closeness. Warmth is as much a frame of mind as a skill and perhaps one developed through being honest with yourself and being prepared to be open with others. It also involves treating the other person as an equal human being.

Martin Buber (1958), the philosopher and therapist, made a distinction between the I–It relationship and the I–Thou (or I–You) relationship. In the I–It relationship, one person treats the other as an object, as a thing. In the I–Thou relationship there occurs a meeting of persons, transcending any differences there may be in terms of status, background, lifestyle, belief or value systems. In the I–Thou relationship there is a sense of sharing and of mutuality, a sense that can be contagious and is of particular value in nursing.

What is not clear is the degree to which a nurse–patient relationship *can* be a mutual relationship. Rogers (1967) argues that the relationship can be a mutual one but Buber acknowledges that because it is always the client who seeks out the professional and comes to that professional with problems, the relationship is, necessarily, unequal and lacking in mutuality. For Buber, the professional relationship starts and progresses from an unequal footing:

> He comes for help to you. You don't come for help to him. And not only this, but you are able, more or less to help him ... You are, of course, a very important person for him. But not a person whom he wants to see and to know and is able to. He is floundering around, he comes to you. He is, may I say, entangled in your life, in your thoughts, in your being, your communication, and so on. But he is not interested in you as you. It cannot be. (Buber, 1965)

Thus warmth must be offered by the nurse but the feeling may not necessarily be reciprocated by the client. There is, as well, another problem with the notion of warmth. We all perceive personal qualities in different sorts of ways. One person's warmth is another person's sickliness or sentimentality. We cannot guarantee how our 'warmth' will be perceived by the other person. In a more general way, however, 'warmth' may be compared to 'coldness'. It is clear that the 'cold' person would not be the ideal person to undertake helping another person in a nursing setting! It is salutary, however, to reflect on the degree to which there are 'cold' people working in the nursing arena and to question why this may be so. It is possible that interpersonal skills training may help this situation for it may be that some 'cold' people are unaware of their coldness.

To a degree, however, our relationships with others tend to be self-monitoring. To a degree, we anticipate, as we go on with a relationship, the effect we are having on others and modify our presentation of self accordingly. Thus we soon get to know if our 'warmth' is too much for the patient or colleague or is being perceived by him in a negative way. This ability to constantly monitor ourselves and our relationships is an important part of the process of developing interpersonal and counselling skills.

Genuineness, too, is another important aspect of the relationship. In one sense, the issue is black or white. We either genuinely care for the person in front of us or we do not. We cannot easily fake professional interest. We must be interested. Some people, however, will interest us more than others. Often, those clients who remind us of our own problems or our own personalities will interest us most of all. This is not so important as our having a genuine interest in the fact that the relationship is happening at all.

On the surface of it, there may appear to be a conflict between the concept of genuineness and the self-monitoring alluded to, above. Self-monitoring may be thought of as 'artificial' or contrived and therefore not genuine. The 'genuineness', discussed here, relates to the nursing professional's interest in the human relationship that is developing between the two people. Any ways in which that relationship can be enhanced must serve a valuable purpose. It is quite possible to be 'genuine' and yet aware of what is happening: genuine and yet committed to increasing interpersonal competence.

Empathic understanding

> 'First of all,' he said, 'if you can learn a simple trick, Scout, you'll get along a lot better with all kinds of folks. You never really understand a person until you consider things from his point of view ...'
>
> 'Sir?'
>
> '... until you climb into his skin and walk around in it.'
>
> (*To Kill a Mockingbird*, Lee, 1960)

Empathy is a relatively new term, apparently coined by Titchner in 1909 to translate the German term *Einfühlung* (Bateson and Coke, 1981). The term is usually used to convey the idea of the ability to enter the perceptual world of the other person: to see the world as they see it. It also suggests an ability to convey this perception to the other person. Kalisch (1971) defines empathy as 'the ability to perceive accurately the feelings of another person and to communicate this understanding to him'.

Empathy is not the same as sympathy. Sympathy suggests 'feeling sorry' for the other person or, perhaps, identifying with how they feel. If a person sympathizes they imagine themselves as being in the other person's position. With empathy the person tries to imagine how it is to be the other person. Feeling sorry for that person does not really come into it. Being empathic, says Rogers (1967):

> means entering the private perceptual world of the other and becoming thoroughly at home in it. It involves being sensitive, moment to moment, to the changing felt meanings which flow in this other person, to the fear or rage or tenderness or confusion or whatever ...

The process of developing empathy involves something of an act of faith. When we empathize with another person, we cannot know what the outcome of that empathizing will be. If we pre-empt the outcome of our empathizing, we are already not empathizing – we are thinking of solutions and of ways of influencing the client towards a particular goal that we have in mind. The process of empathizing involves entering into the perceptual world of the other person without, necessarily, knowing where that process will lead to.

Developing empathic understanding is the process of exploring the client's world, with the client, neither judging nor necessarily offering advice. Perhaps it can be achieved best through the process of carefully attending and listening to the other person and, perhaps, by use of the skills known as 'reflection' which is discussed in a later chapter of this book. It is also a 'way of being', a disposition towards the client, a willingness to explore the other person's problems and to allow the other person to express themselves fully. Again, as with all aspects of the 'client-centred' approach to caring, the empathic approach is underpinned by the idea that it is the client, in the end, who will find their own way through and will find their own answers to their problems in living. To be empathic is to be a fellow traveller, a friend to the person as they undertake the search. Empathic understanding, then, invokes the notion of 'befriending'.

There are, of course, limitations to the degree to which we can truly empathize. Because we all live in different 'worlds' based on our particular culture, education, physiology, belief systems and so forth, we all view that world slightly differently. Thus, to truly empathize with another person would involve actually becoming that other person! We can, however, strive to get as close to the perceptual world of the other by listening and attending and by suspending judgement. We can also learn to forget ourselves, temporarily, and give ourselves as completely as we can to the other person. There is an interesting paradox involved here.

First, we need self-awareness to enable us to develop empathy. Then we need to forget ourselves in order to truly give our empathic attention to the other person.

Unconditional positive regard

Carl Rogers's phrase 'unconditional positive regard' (Rogers, 1967), conveys a particularly important predisposition towards the client, by the nurse. Rogers also called it 'prizing' or even just 'accepting'. It means that the client is viewed with dignity and valued as a worthwhile and positive human being. The 'unconditional' prefix refers to the idea that such regard is offered without any preconditions. Often in relationships some sort of reciprocity is demanded: I will like you (or love you) as long as you return that liking or loving. Rogers is asking that the feelings that the nursing professional holds for the client should be undemanding and not requiring reciprocation.

There is a suggestion of an inherent 'goodness' within the client, bound up in Rogers's notion of unconditional positive regard. This notion of persons as essentially good can be traced back, at least to Rousseau's *Emile* and is philosophically problematic. Arguably, notions such as 'goodness' and 'badness' are social constructions and to argue that a person is born good or bad is fraught. However, as a practical starting point in the nursing relationship, it seems to be a good idea that we assume an inherent, positive and life-asserting characteristic in the client. It seems difficult to argue otherwise. It would be odd, for instance, to engage in the process of counselling with the view that the person was essentially bad, negative and unlikely to grow or develop!

Unconditional positive regard, then, involves a deep and positive feeling for the other person, perhaps equivalent, in the health professions to what Campbell (1984) has called 'moderated love'. He talks of 'lovers and professors', suggesting that certain professionals profess to love, thus claiming both the ability to be professional and to express altruistic love or disinterested love for others. It is interesting that Campbell seems to be suggesting that nursing professionals can 'professionally care' or even 'professionally love' their clients.

On the other hand, Rogers's view of 'natural goodness' and of accepting, totally, the client's point of view has come under criticism from various commentators. Perhaps the most pointed comes from Geller (1984):

> How can Rogers maintain that this [the human process] is fundamentally good and trustworthy, and that one ought to follow the 'calls' and 'appeals' issuing from it? There is so much disconfirming evidence that one can only wonder how Rogers (or anyone) can hold such a view. To drive this point home, consider the case of the fierce misogynist who has a deep-seated desire to degrade and mutilate women. Surely the last thing we would want such a person to do is to act in accordance with his true feelings and desires.

Masson (1988), in a well-known critique of *all* forms of counselling and psychotherapy, offers this view:

What guarantee is there, what guarantee could there possibly be that any given therapist is this genuine person Rogers posits him to be? The unconditional positive regard that Rogers wants the therapist to feel is something that cannot be legislated into existence any more than can be love ... 'Unconditional regard' is not something that seems either likely or desirable. Faced with a brutal rapist who murders children, why should any therapist have unconditional regard for him?

Unconditional positive regard is perhaps the most debatable of Rogers's conditions for effective counselling.

With these caveats in mind, these are the personal qualities that the literature identifies as an important aspect of the counselling relationship. An interesting question is the degree to which such personal qualities can be *learned*. Masson clearly thinks that they cannot. It is perhaps likely that most of us start of with a disposition towards such qualities and that such a disposition can be enhanced by the person paying attention to developing it. Certainly, counselling can never be an automatic, machine-like process. We cannot simply turn on our counselling skills.

On the other hand, neither can we only depend upon having the required personal qualities. If that were so, a lot of people would never even attempt to be nurses or counsellors! The secret lies, perhaps, in combining personal qualities with certain, definable counselling skills. It is here, however that another paradox lies. Can we develop usable counselling skills that we have practised in the presence of our colleagues and friends and still maintain a naturalness and spontaneity – a personal style? Certainly we can. It is worth considering, for a moment, a three-stage model of interpersonal or counselling skills training (Figure 6.1).

Stage One: Individuals are unaware of the range of interpersonal and counselling skills available to them. If they do encounter such a range, they are likely to see the use of such frameworks as 'unnatural' or 'artificial'. This is the person who will argue that counsellors and communicators are born rather than made.

↓

Stage Two: Individuals attend a course or a workshop and explore a range of counselling skills. At this point, because they are *thinking* about what they are doing in their relationships with others, they temporarily become clumsy and awkward.

↓

Stage Three: Individuals have come to incorporate the new skills into their own repertoire. The person is both 'skilled' and 'natural'.

Figure 6.1   A three-stage model of the development of interpersonal and counselling skills

The model is fairly self-explanatory. The person who is new to inter-personal and counselling skills training may be threatened or dismissive of it. As that person comes to learn more about such training, she (or he) begins to experiment with new skills and temporarily becomes *deskilled*. As she progresses, she gradually incorporates the new skills into her own personal style. She is no longer awkward nor a clone of other people. She has developed her own therapeutic style.

Counselling skills in nursing

It is helpful to divide the skills of counselling into two groups:

- Listening and attending; and
- Counselling interventions.

The exercises described in this chapter are aimed at developing both these groups of skills. The exercises may be worked through systematically or individual exercises may be singled out to explore a particular skill.

In order to place these two groups of skills in context, a map of the counselling process is offered in Figure 6.2. In stage one, the counsellor and client meet and gradually come to know each other. This stage may be seen as paralleling the first stage of the nurse–patient relationship.

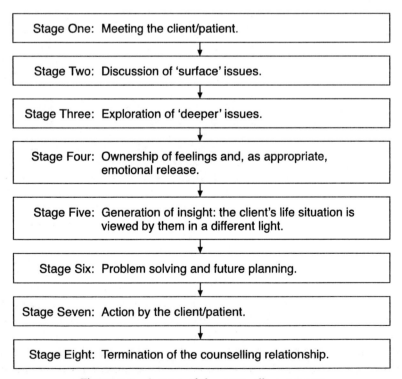

Figure 6.2   A map of the counselling process

Often it is a thawing out process for both the counsellor (or the nurse) and the client (or the patient).

As the counsellor–client or nurse–patient relationship develops the client slowly tests the boundaries of the relationship through discussion of safe, surface issues. Then as trust develops, the topic slowly shifts to deeper existential issues (or to the person's 'deeper' problems). At this stage, the client often realizes the depth of feeling that she has about particular issues: emotional release may occur through the shedding of tears, the expression of anger or through embarrassed laughter. Such a release is known as catharsis and the counsellor or nurse can develop the skills required in helping a person through the process of cathartic release. Such release often enables clients to develop new insights into their condition. It is as though the tears or anger clear away a veil which covers possible solutions to problems or new ways of looking at life issues. Reflection on those new insights can lead to problem-solving or future planning. Such a stage is an important one. Cathartic release, on its own, is not sufficient. Counselling, if it is to help, must be a practical activity. Therefore, the person being counselled needs to be able to plan out what they will do with the insights gained from the emotional release.

Once plans have been made, perhaps through the medium of the counselling or nursing relationship, the client will want to act on those plans. Thus, stage 7, the action stage, takes place away from the counsellor–client relationship and in the client's life situation. Problems, in the end, are not solved by sitting and talking but rather by action. It is the relationship prior to this action that has enabled the action to occur. During this stage, the counsellor's role may only be a supportive one.

Finally, as the client develops more and more autonomy and self-direction, he will need the help of the counsellor or nurse less and less. The time comes when the counselling relationship needs to be terminated and the client and counsellor part. This will often raise all sorts of issues about dependency and independence both in the counsellor and the client. The nurse who is undertaking a lot of counselling needs to explore how she feels about partings and about saying goodbye. Stop reading for a moment and consider what it would feel like to say goodbye to someone close to you. Notice the thoughts and feelings that are brought to the surface by such an idea. Now consider what it may be like for the client who has spent a fair amount of time sharing himself with another person and getting to know that person well. Consider, now, how best you can handle such situations, both from the point of view of *you* as counsellor and of the client.

The map of events described here is an over-simplification. Human relationships are rarely as clear-cut as this. The map does, however, offer some signposts for the direction that the counselling relationship may take. All the stages in the map are also stages in the nurse–patient relationship, although the depth of that relationship will depend upon the needs of the particular patient and the skills of the particular nurse. It is worth bearing in mind that it should always be the client or patient who determines the rate at which the relationship develops. It is, after all, the *client or patient's relationship.* It is not the counsellor or nurse's role to probe, interrogate or in any way force disclosure. Such disclosure, if it is to be therapeutic, must be offered freely by the client or patient and with their goodwill.

Tschudin (1991) offers another way of structuring the counselling relationship through a series of four questions:

1. What is happening?
2. What is the meaning of it?
3. What is your goal?
4. How are you going to do it?

Tschudin suggests that these questions can help the counsellor to keep on track, to offer some structure to what could be a very meandering and structure-less process. The value of the questions is that they are open-ended and can be interpreted variously by both the client and the counsellor.

Counselling skills

The skills described here are ones that can be useful in a wide range of nursing situations, from helping the bereaved person, to counselling colleagues and friends, to helping people who have just received bad news. Perhaps the most important feature to remember when using counselling skills is *timing*. It is not simply a case of learning a set of skills and then using them in counselling situations. Like most things in life, knowing *when* to say something and when to stay silent is most important. It is worth noting what a seventeenth-century writer had to say on this issue, for his words fit the counselling situation almost exactly:

> There is timing in everything. Timing in strategy cannot be mastered without a great deal of practice ... From the outset you must know the applicable timing and the inapplicable timing, and from among the large and small things and the fast and slow timings find the relevant timing, first seeing the distance timing and the background timing. This is the main strategy. It is especially important to know the background timing, otherwise your strategy will become uncertain. (Musashi, 1645)

Understanding of the 'background timing' of counselling is essential and something that, as Musashi suggests, is only learned through a good deal of practice. Counselling skills are never learned simply though attendance at a counselling workshop or even on a one- or two-year certificate or diploma course. The *real* learning takes place in the face-to-face interaction between nurse and patient or client and counsellor.

Counselling and psychotherapy: exploring the differences

Counselling is sometimes compared and confused with psychotherapy. To explore the issues of counselling and psychotherapy as aspects of interpersonal skills in the health care professions, I sought the views of a small group of health professionals who fulfilled either or both of the following criteria: (a) they were trained counsellors *and* health professionals or (b) they taught counselling skills *to* health professionals.

Six health professionals who fulfilled one or both of the above criteria were invited to take part in in-depth interviews with the writer. The sample was a purposive one. Purposive sampling is a non-probability sampling method and one in which the respondents are chosen for the study according to the likelihood of their being able to talk on the topic in hand. If a researcher is exploring counselling with health care professionals then it is appropriate that 'health care professionals' become the population from which that sample is drawn.

Although a range of ideas and topics were covered in these interviews it is unlikely that data saturation occurred. Also, no attempt is being made to generalize these findings. In common with other small-scale qualitative studies, the aim is to illuminate and to offer ideas for discussion and further work.

Interviews were conducted using a semi-structured interview schedule. In a semi-structured interview, certain *topics* are always alluded to in each interview but the *ordering* and *form* of the questions does not necessarily remain the same. This approach to interviewing allows the interview to progress in a fairly spontaneous manner and allows for the interviewer to 'follow' rather than 'lead' the respondent.

The interviews were transcribed and then content-analysed into a series of themes. What follows is an elaboration of the findings accompanied by some commentary on the responses. The aim was to explore the data and to organize them according to emergent themes. These themes were partly dictated by the semi-structured interview schedule and partly through combing through the data and noting particular issues that were discussed by respondents.

Definition of counselling

Respondents offered various definitions of counselling. Sometimes, those definitions referred to the *purpose or application* of counselling:

> I think that [counselling] is any kind of assistance in helping people to come to terms with an emotional or spiritual problem of any kind. It is not confined to mental distress or mental disorder. It can range from things like being in debt to having acute depression.

Another respondent offered much more of a 'textbook' definition and followed this up by suggesting some of the purposes of counselling.

> Counselling is an activity in which one person is helping and one is receiving help and in which the emphasis of that help is on enabling the other person to find solutions to problems or to look at particular situations which they would like resolved. Or to enable them to live more resourcefully. It involves the development, by the counsellor, of a range of particular skills but more importantly the adoption of a particular stance or attitude towards the person being helped and that includes the person feeling valued and able to explore

the way in which he perceives himself and his world and not to feel judged by the counsellor.

Yet another hinted at a 'contract' but was not clear on this issue. However, as we shall see, some respondents *did* feel that counselling was contractual.

> I think counselling is an activity in which two people agree to meet under certain conditions. And these conditions may be overt and negotiated and include such issues as confidentiality and expected outcomes. It is very much an interpersonal activity and the counsellor is there to help the client address and possibly resolve issues that are personal and meaningful to that individual.

One respondent referred to the need for the counsellor to remain *ordinary*. The argument is that other people are likely to respond to us more readily if we do not attempt to assume a 'professional' front or one that is 'artificial' in any way.

> For me, it is a means of just being with another person who may need to talk over problems, job difficulties, personal dilemmas and so forth. In much the same way as you talk things over with a spouse or friend. That *ordinariness*, if you like, is important in counselling.

Another respondent discussed counselling in terms of 'helping people to help themselves' – a point that the respondent felt was echoed in the literature on the topic:

> Counselling is creating an environment in which people can explore the issues – whatever they are, whether it is a particular way of looking at life, a childhood issue, perhaps – in a supportive atmosphere. One official definition is 'helping people to help themselves' and I quite like that: I think it's a good synopsis.

Counselling and psychotherapy

As we have seen from the discussion above, there is plenty of contention about what does or does not differentiate counselling from psychotherapy. This contention was mirrored in the responses from respondents in the study.

> Psychotherapy specifically applies to a clinical and mental illness as opposed to the neuroses that run through society. Psychotherapy is done by psychotherapists (as opposed to counsellors) and who can be lay therapists or qualified ones. Whereas counselling can be done by a whole range of people, from priests to professional counsellors.

> I would guess that counselling would have a much more practical, every day, problem-solving slant to it – grounded in the here-and-now. Whereas psychotherapy, for me, evokes ideas to do with Freudian psychology ...

Another respondent hinted at the Freudian approach to psychotherapy without making the issue explicit.

> I would see psychotherapy as exploring the person's life at a much deeper level, including the development of insight based on exploration of early

development, parental influences and those things *may* come into counselling. In counselling they are brought in to understand a *particular* situation rather than to understand the client him or herself.

The idea of the 'here-and-now' arose in another respondents' interview:

> I perceive psychotherapy as being different in a variety of areas. Psychotherapists tend to be educated and trained within a particular school of practice. They tend to be in therapy themselves as part of their training. And they would claim to work with individuals at a greater depth. I see them working more in the 'there and then' than the 'here and now' ... The term is bound up with certain political issues – such as it is seen as more complex and goes on for longer and entails perhaps greater exploration and commitment on the part of the client.

One respondent had personal experience of *both* counselling and psychotherapy and made few distinctions between them. This may be a particularly important contribution to the debate given that it comes from someone who has had first-hand experience of both sorts of 'therapy'.

> I've had both psychotherapy and counselling as part of my on-going training. I can't say there seems to be that much difference. Some see psychotherapy as synonymous with psychoanalysis but I find it difficult to make that distinction. Counselling doesn't go as deep as psychotherapy. Psychotherapy is a bit of a status thing as well. But there are other sorts of psychotherapy – TA [transactional analysis] and so on. I don't know really, the distinctions are blurred.

What the 'status thing' was is not made clear in the interview and was not pursued by the interviewer. The respondent *seems* to be hinting at the idea that having psychotherapy may be viewed as engaging in a 'higher status' activity than would be the case with having counselling.

Counselling and other sorts of conversation

If there were conflicting reports about what counselling and psychotherapy were, then it seemed reasonable to try to define the boundaries of counselling in another way. To this end, respondents were asked what the differences were between counselling and *other* sorts of conversation. If counselling is a discrete activity (as opposed to, for example, simply talking things over with a friend), then it seems reasonable that those who do it should be able to distinguish between simply 'talking' about something and 'doing counselling'. One respondent saw the difference in terms of *structure* – the counselling relationship was a more structured one than the more informal conversation:

> The only difference that I can see is in their formal structure. If things can be achieved by talking to your friends in the pub then that's fine. Whereas counselling usually has some sort of formal structure involved. It is also a professional relationship in the sense of a counsellor and client where the counsellor is paid to counsel or listen.

It should be noted that the previous respondent viewed counselling as an activity that was paid for by the client. Other respondents described the differences in terms of the *roles* played out by the participants in counselling:

> In counselling you would expect that one of the people has a problem, a dilemma that they are facing and that tends to be the focus of the interaction. Whereas the other person is seen as a counsellor, helper or listener. In a normal conversation that state of affairs might apply but it might also not apply and there may just be small talk about any aspect of the person's life. If you build on that definitional difference the more professional the counsellor, or the more formalized the counselling, the greater the difference would be between the helper and the helpee in terms of power, status and so forth. For example, if I go along to a friend of mine and talk about work or home problems, I won't feel guarded about status or power or being exposed psychologically because in that relationship it is guided by the principles of friendship or collegial relationships. On the other hand, if I found that I had to attend a marriage guidance counsellor, for example, I would find that rather uncomfortable. At least to begin with. And I would be very aware that I was the one with the problem and that he or she would be the person with the fix-it solution.

One is in the allocation of roles. That is the roles of helper and helpee. I think the specific aims of the conversation are to help. It is purposeful and directed towards helping and a counsellor has no other motives other than to help. People have argued that one of the differences is that the more therapeutic a conversation is, the more likely it is to acknowledge what is happening in the here and now – in this relationship. It will include an emphasis on recognizing feelings as well as thoughts. This is not to imply that ordinary conversation can't be altruistic. Egan's language of saying 'helping' and of what he calls 'helping' and we would call 'counselling' emphasizes this idea that counselling is helping.

For another respondent, the two types of interaction were often blurred. It was sometimes difficult to say what the difference was between counselling and 'ordinary conversation':

> I think that it is a difficult question because sometimes an ordinary conversation turns into counselling and a counsellor may use counselling skills in their conversational life. I also think that counselling skills can enhance conversation and perhaps, thinking as we talk about this, counselling is a specific form of conversation. I think sometimes the differences can be small and that initial sessions of clients can be 'conversational'. But they move into a counselling arena. I suspect that conversation is more reciprocal in depth and content whereas counselling tends to be less so – particularly on the part of the counsellor.

On the other hand, another respondent was very clear about the differences and saw them in *contractual* terms:

> Counselling has very specific parameters. There is a contract, you know how long you will meet and so on. It is a very specific type of conversation. And although some of the skills and things the counsellor may be demonstrating are similar to other conversations it is very *intentional*. It is not two-way as in other conversations. The focus in counselling is very much on the client. It is intentional-focused.

What this respondent did not spell out was whether he felt that the contract was *implicit* rather than *explicit*. Presumably few counsellors or their clients draw up formal contracts. If, on the other hand, the contract is an *implicit* one, the question is raised as to whether the client fully understands the 'rules of the contract'.

Who does counselling?

If counselling is something to be considered as a therapeutic option by health professionals, it is important to know what sorts of people *do* counselling. Should they be *qualified*? Should they be 'professionals' and so on. There were various responses to this sort of question.

> Essentially anyone can do counselling. But for the most part it tends to be either professional counsellors or people who have traditionally had a counselling role, such as doctors, nurses or priests.

People do counselling who are interested in other people and who are prepared to spend time with them, supporting them. Anyone could, in that respect, do counselling. Whereas in the more formal type of counselling, the formal helping agencies, you get the doctors, the social workers, the lawyers, the bar tenders. Then there are the people who set themselves up as professional counsellors. I don't know people who work like that but I guess they exist.

I think that counselling could be done by anyone but is more likely to be done better by someone who has had the opportunity to develop specific skills and who has been able to explore some of his characteristics and things like warmth, genuineness etc. However, it is likely that many people already possess those qualities and therefore will be better helpers than people who do not. I think there is a danger in saying that counselling is the preserve of counsellors because that relates it directly to training and I am not sure there is any evidence to demonstrate that training really does make a difference.

One respondent made a distinction between those who do counselling as part of another professional role and those who do it as a full-time job.

> I would argue that there is a range of professionals whose primary professional role is working with people, such as teaching, social work, nursing, medicine, and in which the aim is to help others and where often that help is given through the medium of some sort of personal interaction. The more that interaction is the sole means of helping then the more we move towards that situation being counselling. For example, in medicine we see the prescribing of treatment and the relationship is not the sole means of helping. Clearly, there are some whose role is only seen as counselling and who have no other agenda. They do not have an educational agenda, a teaching agenda – the work they do is whatever the client brings. We can say then that they have a 'pure' counselling role.

Another respondent added a little to the confusion of the issues by offering a tautological response to the question of 'who counsels?' The same respondent, however, also indicates – at least, laterally – that many people *could* do counselling – those who were considered 'wise' and those, presumably, who had sufficient and appropriate life experience.

> Counsellors do counselling! Counsellors also teach other people counselling skills in the belief that it enhances communication. I think perhaps counselling can be an unrecognized ability of those who are considered wise and of whom there aren't enough.

Most of the above respondents took the 'anyone can do counselling' approach. Others, however, wanted counselling to be more formalized and for counsellors to be trained

> People who [do counselling] are qualified counsellors. Although there may be people who have not done a proper certificate or diploma but who do counsel from experience. There are elements of counselling and counselling skills that occur in a lot of caring conversations that are carried out by health care professionals. It would be wrong to 'counsel' somebody without their permission and without a contract because of counselling's potential power.

How counselling can be used

If counselling is a therapeutic activity, it seems important to know what sorts of things counselling can be used for. These respondents were drawn from a number of sources within the transcripts.

> There are a whole range of practical difficulties that can be helped by counselling, such as difficulty with study skills and getting into higher education, through to things like depression following bereavement, or neuroses or mental illnesses. There has been an expansion in the profession of counselling in recent years – you often get the situation where someone calls themselves a professional counsellor on the basis of a range of qualifications that carry no guarantee as to the likely effectiveness of that counselling. At the same time, people with a lot of experience – such as psychiatric nurses – would not, necessarily, have that qualification recognized as appropriate in counselling. I think there is a process of excluding people from counselling as an occupation going on, which is similar to the way in which health professionals exclude other people from working in health care – so that health care adopted a professional strategy for excluding people and counselling is doing the same. Counselling is becoming a workplace strategy which has the interest of the counsellor at heart and not necessarily those of the clients. The role of the qualification in counselling is exclusion rather than testing professional competence. You could have a very competent counsellor who is competent on the basis of their qualities but that would allow any number of people to become counsellors, which would disrupt the professional aspirations of a lot of counsellors.

One respondent discussed the use of counselling in terms of its *structure* and how little or much the counselling relationship needed to be structured:

It can be used on a daily basis or on an informal basis with contacts with colleagues and people you are attached to. I guess this is the more informal type of counselling. Then there are the more professional settings – tutors to students for example, when you have to make yourself approachable to the students. That needs a little bit more thought. Some of the people who are tutors are there for academic tutoring, others are there for all aspects of the student's life. Perhaps a middle path is necessary here: where tutors are prepared to listen to what is going on outside the student's immediate academic arena.

Another talked of 'formalized' counselling (as opposed, presumably, to informal or 'friendly' counselling). He noted, too, some possible *arenas* for counselling.

There is the more highly formalized counselling situation – counselling people, getting paid to do it, perhaps being part of a team helping GPs, psychiatrists etc. You may be a practitioner in a psychiatric unit or other care setting. All of these different situations are ones in which some form of counselling might be called for.

Another respondent made this distinction between 'formal' and 'informal' approaches to counselling more explicit:

There are at least two types of counselling: the informal, ordinary, unspectacular way of helping and the more professional side of things. I find that the phoniness you meet sometimes – the tilted head, the voice changing – may be a result of the training. I find that off-putting. What I need when I discuss something with somebody else is a gut reaction – a more spontaneous reaction. I would not approach a stranger for that. I would need to know the person was genuinely interested in me.

Yet another respondent talked of the difficulty of training counsellors and of the paradox between 'being spontaneous' and 'being a professional':

The spontaneous part of counselling is *very* difficult to train at all. It has to do with people knowing their limitations and their likes and dislikes. As you professionalize something there is the tendency to make things more special, more detached from the real side of a relationship. Something gets lost. There is a risk of losing the spontaneous side of the interaction.

Others saw the value of counselling as lying within the process of helping people to become more responsible for themselves and re-exercising some control over what happens to them:

It can be used to enable people to examine specific problems or life situations which they would like resolved or changed. To enable them to make the best use of resources, to examine relationships, to make choices, to discover the choices available to them. To help them become more responsible for themselves and to use that responsibility over their own lives. To enable them to feel more in control of their situation. To enable them to be in a relationship with a counsellor which will enable them to develop learnings about themselves. And to make those discoveries in a situation which, although it may be uncomfortable, is safe.

It can be used to enable people to problem-solve, to identify sources of discomfort or stress and it can be used to alleviate problems of living – everyday problems of living such as anxiety and general feelings that people have of being 'outside'. It can also enhance basic communication. It can also be used, perhaps inappropriately. It can be used as a disguise for basic disciplinary measures and it can be hi-jacked to disguise commercial activities such as beauty counsellors, financial counsellors etc.

Some respondents felt there was a tension between health professionals offering counselling and counselling being viewed as a 'treatment'. It was seen as essential that becoming involved in counselling should be a voluntary activity on the part of the patient or client.

> I don't think there is ever a 'should' – 'this person should see a counsellor'. If they are not ready and they don't want it, then there is no point. I very much believe in people's rights to live their own life the way they want and not have counselling. When somebody is going through a traumatic experience then there are all sorts of problems that are unresolved, particularly when they do not have other people in their lives to talk to. Even when people do have lots of other people counselling is quite different. Family and friends will not talk to you in the same way. Counsellors are impartial and will not necessarily just go with you. Friends will not want to upset you whereas counselling can be more penetrating and challenging – which friends will not always be – unless they are special friends. Any sorts of problems – mid-life crises, 'what's it all about' – those sorts of issues can be addressed in counselling.

When counselling should not be used

Respondents talked about when counselling *should not* be used – contra-indications of counselling. These were wide-ranging and are reported below. The first seems to relate to the misuse of certain sorts of training procedures.

> It shouldn't be used as a habit or for recreational purposes. I have seen some people who seem to be addicted to it. It becomes a substitution for normal human intercourse and sometimes people's motives are poor for going into it in the first place – such as group counselling as a place to pick up women.

> There may be a danger that a vulnerable person could be exposed psychologic-ally or abused – using the term broadly. If you were, for example, attracted to a person of the opposite sex, or the same sex, that may infect the situation if you had a lot of contact with them. As a counsellor you need to be pretty solid, you need to know what you are doing and your integrity is not going to be called into question. You have to be seen as being detached but that's not a word that rests easy, you have to be comfortable in your own skin – whatever people say to you, you're not going to be tempted to abuse the relationship. Those things relate more to the professional dimension than to the ordinary side.

Sometimes, the issue was an ideological one. It was noted by one respondent that the prevailing philosophy in counselling is the 'client-centred' one in which the client is *always* encouraged to find his or her own solutions to his or her problems and in which direct, prescriptive intervention on the part of the client is usually eschewed.

It may depend on the type of counselling the counsellor wishes to adopt. To adopt a non-directive approach with people where it is patently obvious that you should be making suggestions, is very wasteful, I think there are lots of people who seek out help who want a direction and to keep throwing back on them and ask them to make every decision is sometimes inappropriate. People are pretty good at problem-solving and are likely to respond much better to the non-directive approach but there are people who find it difficult to make any decisions and then it is appropriate to make more concrete suggestions as to what they may do.

Sometimes, the fact that counselling was not a panacea was noted and it was made clear that counselling had very definite limitations. The following respondents highlight the problems of the then current practice of counsellors to be 'to hand' after a major disaster.

There may be situations where the problem cannot be solved in your head – and I'm thinking about lack of money, serious illness, unemployment – those sorts of things. Counselling may help but some of those very serious problems aren't ones that can be solved. Or these emergency situations that we see on the TV – kids drowning, accidents and things – its amazing how quickly counselling services are set up. And yet what most normal people would be is in a state of shock at that time, and its seems likely that only afterwards people need counselling – not immediately afterwards. I can't see how anyone can sit in an aircraft hangar and have twenty counsellors dashing towards them. You have the same sort of situation when children have been murdered or have disappeared and you have loads of counsellors dashing round to the school to these thirteen- or fourteen-year-olds to do counselling, when all they need probably is to be reassured by their parents.

I think I would also disagree with those who feel that the presence of counsellors at disasters is probably inappropriate. You get a vision of 'therapeutic vultures' perhaps when people are in a extreme distress they need time to be distressed. Because counselling is not a universal panacea for the human condition.

Sometimes, the client-centred approach, referred to above, was seen as limited and one respondent called for a much wider approach to be used:

When the counsellor has other motives other than to help the client: when the counsellor is in a situation which he himself ought to take responsibility for the situation, either because of former responsibilities for it or when not to do so would cause undue pain to the client – such as when you look at situations in which people steadfastly avoid giving advice by trying to be Rogerian – when the best thing would be to tell the person what to do. I recognize that in counselling you would tend to avoid that but sometimes it would be more appropriate. I think John Heron's material on prescriptive and informative interventions is quite helpful in that way.

The question of the counsellor's 'detachment' was another issue that was discussed by some of the respondents. The issue of 'boundaries' was also discussed:

I think that where there is another relationship in which it is impossible for the counsellor to be detached – . . . relatives, that sort of thing. That is not to imply you can never help people close to you because I think you can. It's just that there's a way of being in counselling which is not appropriate to close relationships, family or sex relationships. I think it is about boundaries in counselling so that it would be inappropriate for me to take on a student for counselling in its pure sense where I also had another relationship where I also judged the students. That is not to say that I cannot help the students but that I would not take them on for a review of their personal life situation and would recommend that they get their help from someone else.

There are real problems when the client doesn't want counselling. In fact when the individual does not want to be a client. This is a particular problem of people on counselling courses who insist on asking people 'how they feel'. It should not be used as a crowbar for intruding into people's privacy.

The advantages of counselling

Various advantages of counselling were identified by the respondents. One respondent identified its *economic* advantages. He also referred, in passing, to the role of the Church in counselling and the idea of 'counselling as a replacement for a priest'.

It can help you over an immediate crisis or problem. If you are upset you often can't see a way out of a predicament. It's a cheap relative to psychoanalysis or psychotherapy. It is also widely available. A counsellor will give you time in a way that a doctor won't. And for an atheist like myself, a priest is not really an alternative. For a religious person, a priest may be the most appropriate person as the problem may have a spiritual content.

Others found other advantages but often these were *qualified* in various ways suggesting that with the various advantages also came other disadvantages:

My guess is that it helps people just to get on with their lives. The fact that I think lots of people can do it. But it does need a willingness and a genuine interest in other human beings which is difficult to 'manufacture'. It can be pretty cheap – a cheap way of helping people. The less formal types of counselling perhaps allow the person who needs the help to maintain some dignity and integrity in the whole process and its not like going to your doctor or going to a psychiatrist because your whole life is falling apart – its sort of more acceptable to society. You can say to people 'I'm going for some counselling' but it is more difficult to say 'I was mentally ill'. There is a greater willingness for people to take counselling on board as acceptable.

[Counselling helps people to have] the opportunity to have a safe situation in which one explores options and choices – particularly where some of those choices may be frightening or where some disclosures of some aspects of one's self may be a presentation of self that one wouldn't want seen elsewhere. If I am looking at a side of myself that I don't want to show to people in everyday life but I need to understand, then I may need the confidentiality of a counselling relationship in order to do that.

Sometimes, the view was taken that 'counselling works because people say that it does':

> For the client it would seem to help. I am not sure why. Perhaps I am a bit but it seems to help. I've seen it help. And sometimes afterwards I've wondered what I've done that I valued so much and that I missed. I guess that relates to the intuitive nature of counselling if you have counselled for a while.

The disadvantages of counselling

There were also clearly identified *disadvantages* to counselling. Again, these were quite wide-ranging.

> It can mislead people into thinking it's a solution, when in fact a real solution may be a material change in the person's circumstances which the counsellor can do nothing to effect. There are a lot of charlatans in counselling. When there is money changing hands the counsellors may have more interest in prolonging the sessions. It is a straightforward market relation sometimes. And like all market relations the profit is a motive and not a human need. The other thing is it is just another way of accommodating oneself to what may be a horrible situation and a better response may be a political one.

One respondent had doubts about the purported practice of teaching student health professionals counselling skills as part of their health care training – arguing that counsellors needed some maturity and some life experience in order to both help the client and to take care of themselves:

> One of the things which is true about counselling is that is has become reified – it has become elevated to a supernatural status – particularly in health care. So much so that every curriculum document must have an element of counselling in it. My feeling is that many of the students that I have dealt with are anywhere between 17 and 22 and I do believe that if you're going to be a good counsellor you need to have more life experience as it will help you to put things in perspective. It seems that some courses are expecting to put these young people into counselling and turn them out as mini-counsellors in any arena. I don't think that this is realistic and this is one of the problems as the thing has become more popular. So you have people coming out of courses who will I think have done all these hours of counselling training but these are not underpinned by the years of experience that are needed to be a good counsellor.

Other disadvantages were also noted:

> There is the potential opportunity to abuse other people's vulnerability. People do enjoy having power, as experts over people who are very vulnerable and I think this is something to have to guard against.

> I would want to distinguish between bad counselling – which one could find quite easily and which could be disempowering and could produce dependency, could mean the person does not own their own decisions. I think there is a continuum in counselling. As counselling gets better the likelihood of those happening are reduced. The good counsellor with a good supervisor would be careful not to let those things happen and would be aware of their propensities to allow those things to happen and would be aware of their own needs to let them happen. In other words the counsellor who gets a buzz out of

counselling or enjoys being needed or who wants to take credit for other people's successes is likely to make those disadvantages happen. If one develops as a responsible counsellor one tries to avoid those things. I think we should recognize our own propensity to want to be needed but if we are counselling properly we will look out for that happening.

For the client perhaps, they may feel that it doesn't supply them with any answers. The process can be seen as rather slow or even traumatic.

For the counsellor the disadvantages are that it opens you to an awareness of another person's pain that you may have to avoid due to the situation you are in. And perhaps it can make you weary of other people's distress.

Listening and attending

To listen to another person is the most human of actions. In counselling it is the crucial skill. The experiential exercises that follow aim to develop the skill of listening and giving attention. Listening refers to the process of *hearing* what the client is saying. Hearing encompasses not only the words that are being used but also the non-verbal aspects of the encounter. Thus *attending* refers to the counsellor's skill in paying attention to the client, in keeping attention focused 'out' as described in the first chapter.

Why listen? Hargie, Saunders and Dickson (1994) list the general functions of listening as follows:

- to focus specifically upon the messages being communicated by the other person;
- to gain full, accurate understanding of the other person's communication;
- to convey interest, concern and attention;
- to encourage full, open and honest expression;
- to develop and 'other-centred' approach during an interaction.

Throughout all the exercises in this chapter, the words facilitator, counsellor and client are used for convenience. It should be noted that the words tutor (or lecturer), nurse and patient can just as easily be used in their place. The personal pronouns he and she have been used interchangeably.

Once again, the participants in these exercises are exhorted to 'stay awake' whilst doing them. It is vital that the person *notices*: notices her own feelings and thoughts, his own body position, posture, eye contact and so forth. The mystic George Gurdjieff maintained that for most of what we call the waking state, we were, in fact, 'asleep' – we simply did not *notice* (Reyner, 1984). Ouspensky, a follower of Gurdjieff, went on to suggest that we only really learned new things and remembered what has happening to us when we 'stayed awake'. The Christian mystic Simone Weil added a spiritual dimension to the notion of attending when she suggested that true noticing of what was happening around us was an acknowledgement of God (Weill, 1967). Brother Lawrence called noticing and attending 'The Practice of the Presence of God' (Lawrence, 1981).

Thus the topic has been addressed both from secular and spiritual points of view.

The nurse who practises regularly the feat of noticing can become more observant, more sensitive to the needs of others and more self-aware. Indeed, to notice in this way is to be fully present in the moment that is being lived. The first series of exercises concentrates on a variety of aspects of listening and attending.

> If you think back to the coffee shop or picnic table or similar situations you will remember that people are, everywhere and at all times in the presence of each other, either trying to be listened to – taking every chance they get – or waiting impatiently for a chance to interrupt any other person who is talking and start talking themselves. You will find that whenever people are together, they're making an effort to be listened to, and *are* very seldom listened to because the person that they are trying to get to listen to them is waiting, desperately and impatiently for a chance to be listened to himself or herself. (Jackins, 1983)

Exercises in listening and attending

Exercise 1

Aim of the exercise: To enable participants to get attention 'out'.
Group size: Any number from 6 to 20.
Time required: About 20 to 30 minutes.
Materials and/or environment required: A large, comfortable room and a circle of straight-backed chairs.

Process

1. The facilitator invites the group to divide into pairs.
2. Each pair nominates one of them as 'A' and one as 'B'.
3. 'A' then describes in detail for 2 minutes. what 'B' looks like: hair, facial expression, clothing and so on. Such a description should be 'literal' and concrete and free of value judgements.
4. 'B' listens silently to 'A''s description.
5. After 5 minutes the facilitator invites the pairs to exchange roles: thus 'B' describes, literally, 'A''s appearance.
6. When both aspects of the exercise have been completed, the facilitator asks the group to reconvene and encourages feedback with an open question such as 'What happened?'

Evaluation

The facilitator may also want to explore with the group how they *felt* about doing the exercise. She may also encourage group members to describe any problems that they have with the activity.

Notes

A 'solo' version of this activity can be used as a method of paying attention to and describing a person (or an object) outside of oneself as a method of getting attention 'out' prior to talking to a patient or commencing counselling. In this case, it is done silently and alone and is valuable as a means of freshening attention at any time.

Exercise 2

Aim of the exercise: To explore proximity and spatial relationships between two people.
Group size: Any number from 6 to 20.
Time required: About 1 hour.
Materials and/or environment required: A large, comfortable room and a circle of straight-backed chairs.

Process

1. The facilitator asks the group to divide into pairs.
2. Each pair nominates one of them as 'A' and the other as 'B'.
3. 'A' and 'B' then sit about 4 ft apart and hold a conversation.
4. After 5 minutes, 'A' and 'B' move their seats forward until their knees are almost touching and continue the conversation for another 5 minutes.
5. After the second phase of the activity, the facilitator leads a discussion on the issue of space between talker and listener.

Evaluation

The facilitator may want to ask:

- Which was worse, sitting too close or too far away?
- Do you ever stand or sit too close to other people?

Notes

On the subject of proximity, Roger Brown (1965) makes the interesting observation that you can move someone backwards round a room by constantly overstepping the 'right' space between you, by small increments! A curious fact. Try it!

It is important to discuss *cultural* differences in acceptable spaces between people. This is a vital issue when counselling people from different cultures.

Exercise 3

Aim of the exercise: To explore eye contact whilst listening.
Group size: Any number from 6 to 20.
Time required: About 1 hour.
Materials and/or environment required: A large, comfortable room and a circle of straight-backed chairs.

Process

1. The facilitator invites the group to divide into pairs.
2. Each pair nominates one of them as 'A' and one as 'B'.
3. 'A' talks to 'B' on one of the following topics:
   (a) favourite foods
   (b) people I like
   (c) why I want to stay in nursing.
4. During this time, 'A' tries to maintain *constant* eye contact.
5. After 5 minutes, 'A' and 'B' switch roles and 'A' talks to 'B' whilst 'B' maintains *constant* eye contact.

Evaluation

The facilitator may want to ask:

- What did that feel like?
- How do you *know* how much eye contact to make?
- What makes eye contact difficult?

Notes

The notes above about cultural factors apply equally much to the issue of eye contact. It is easy to mismanage the question of eye contact where people from very different cultures are concerned.

Exercise 4

Aim of the exercise: To explore the verbal and non-verbal aspects of listening.
Group size: Any number from 6 to 20.
Time required: About 40 minutes.
Materials and/or environment required: A large, comfortable room and a circle of straight-backed chairs.

Process

1. The facilitator invites the group to divide into pairs.
2. Each pair nominates one of them as 'A' and one as 'B'.

3. 'A' talks to 'B' for 5 minutes on one of the following topics:
   (a) interests away from work
   (b) recent clinical experiences
   (c) past or future holidays.
4. Whilst 'A' is talking, 'B' does NOT listen.
5. After 5 minutes, the facilitator asks the pairs to exchange roles: thus 'B' talks to 'A' and 'A' does not listen.
6. When both aspects of the exercise have been completed, the facilitator invites the group to reconvene and encourages feedback with an open question.

Evaluation

The facilitator may want to explore the following sorts of questions with the group:

- What did it feel like *not* to be listened to?
- What did it feel like to sit and *not* listen to someone?
- What did you do to *avoid* listening?
- What did you do when you realized you could hear what the other person was saying?
- Do you recognize the 'non-listener' from clinical practice?
- How effective is *your* listening ability?

Notes

A variation on this exercise is to have the pairs sitting back-to back, so that 'A' talks to 'B' but cannot see 'B'.

Effective listening behaviours

Following this exercise it is common for a discussion to develop on the importance of non-verbal behaviour when listening to another person or when counselling them. Gerard Egan (1986) offers a useful acronym – SOLER – for remembering the important aspects of non-verbal activity during the listening process. This is illustrated in Figure 6.3.

Egan argues that, in Western countries, these behaviours are usually associated with effective listening. Sitting squarely means sitting opposite the person who is being listened to, rather than next to them. In this way, the one doing the listening can see *all* of the other person and can observe the non-verbal behaviours of the talker. The position also demonstrates interest in the other person.

An open position means that the listener does not have his or her arms crossed. Such crossings can be create real or psychological barriers. The *closed* position can often be construed as being defensive, as we shall see in the next exercise.

Eye contact should be steady and appropriate. No one wants to be stared at but neither do they want to feel that the person who is supposed to be listening to them will look anywhere but at them. As we have noted,

S — Sit *squarely* in relation to the person.
O — Maintain an *open* position.
L — *Lean* slightly towards the other person.
E — Maintain reasonable *eye contact* with them.
R — Try to *relax.*

Figure 6.3 The behavioural aspects of listening (after Egan, 1986)

too, cultural factors play a part in determining how much or how little eye contact may be made. Eye contact may also depend upon the relative status of the pair involved. Finally, the listener should try to sit quietly and be relaxed. T.S. Eliot summed up this position well when he wrote:

Teach us to care and not to care.
Teach us to sit still.

(Eliot, 'Ash-Wednesday', 1930/1963)

When listening to another person, we do not have to be constantly rehearsing what *we* will say next. Nor do we have to relate everything that is said to *us* and to our own thoughts and feelings. The ability to sit and quietly listen may be the greatest of all counselling skills.

Egan's guidelines on how to sit when listening to another person may be useful as a baseline. Clearly, no one wants to talk to a person who sits and looks like a statue! On the other hand, it doesn't help very much to sit, lounge and fidget when listening. The SOLER acronym serves as a gentle reminder and guide whilst listening and counselling. Don't become a slave to it.

Hargie, Saunders and Dickson (1994) offer the following basic guidelines to be borne in mind when listening:

- Get physically prepared to listen ...
- Be mentally prepared to listen objectively ...
- Use spare thought time positively ...
- Avoid interrupting the speaker where possible ...
- Organize the speaker's messages into appropriate categories and, where possible, into chronological order ...
- Don't overuse blocking tactics ...
- Remember that listening is hard work.

Exercise 5

Aim of the exercise: To explore the verbal and non-verbal aspects of listening and giving attention.
Group size: Any number from 6 to 20.
Time required: About 40 minutes.
Materials and/or environment required: A large, comfortable room and a circle of straight-backed chairs.

Process

1. The facilitator asks the group to divide into pairs.
2. Each pair nominates one of them as 'A' and one as 'B'.
3. 'A' talks to 'B' for 5 minutes on one of the following topics:
   (a) the future of nursing
   (b) problems of training
   (c) music and/or books that I like.
4. 'B' *contradicts* the first four SOLER behaviours described in the text. In other words, he:
   (a) does *not* sit squarely to the other person but sits next to her instead
   (b) maintains a *closed* position with arms and legs crossed
   (c) leans *away* from the other person, rather than *towards* her
   (d) makes *no* eye contact with the other person ... BUT *listens to* 'A'!
5. After 5 minutes, roles are reversed and 'B' talks to 'A', whilst 'A' contradicts the first four SOLER behaviours.
6. When both aspects of the exercises have been completed, the facilitator reconvenes the group and leads a discussion about what happened.

Evaluation

The facilitator may want to ask:

- What did it feel like to be listened to by someone who *did not appear* to be listening to you?
- What was it like *not* to demonstrate that you were listening?
- What does all this say about your own listening?

Notes

The facilitator is advised to suggest to the group that they do not over-dramatize the contradictions of the SOLER behaviours and also to emphasize the fact that group members are to LISTEN to each other. This last fact tends to get forgotten when the behaviours are contradicted!

Minimal prompts

For this and other exercises, group members may find the use of 'minimal prompts' helpful. Figure 6.4 offers examples of such prompts. The aim is to become familiar with the range of possible prompts available and to use them knowingly and out of choice. Often our behaviour becomes so automatic that we do not notice the minimal prompts that we use in everyday conversation. Exercises of this sort can help to encourage people to make conscious decisions about their use of such prompts.

Exercise 6

Aim of the exercise: To explore the use of minimal prompts.
Group size: Any number from 6 to 20.

Examples of verbal prompts:

'Yes'
'OK'
'Go on . . .'
'Ah-ha'
'Mm . . .'
'Right'
'I see . . .'

Examples of non-verbal prompts:

Head nods
Smiles
Raised eyebrows
Encouraging hand movements
Gentle touch

Figure 6.4   Examples of minimal prompts in listening

Time required: About 40 minutes to 1 hour.
Materials and/or environment required: A large, comfortable room and a circle of straight-backed chairs.

Process

1. The facilitator invites the group to divide into pairs.
2. Each pair nominates one of them as 'A' and one as 'B'.
3. 'A' talks to 'B' for 5 minutes about one of the following topics:
   (a) the sort of person that I would like to be
   (b) my skills as a nurse
   (c) what I would do if I had a million pounds.
4. 'B' listens but uses *exaggerated* minimal prompts and does not talk or respond to 'B' in any other way.
5. After 5 minutes, roles are reversed and 'B' talks to 'A', whilst 'A' uses exaggerated minimal prompts.
6. When both parts of the exercise have been completed, the group is reconvened and the facilitator leads a discussion on what happened.

Evaluation

The facilitator may like to ask the group:

- What were you reminded of when you did this exercise?
- Are you ever *normally* like this?
- Were you reminded of anyone else when you did this activity?
- What are the problems of overuse of minimal prompts?

Notes

This exercise is an example of what may be called exaggerated negative role play. Practising *poor* examples of counselling skills can be a powerful way of encouraging *good* practice. Activities of this sort can cause much hilarity on the part of the participants!

Exercise 7

Aim of the exercise: To practise listening and giving attention with appropriate verbal and non-verbal behaviours.
Group size: Any number from 6 to 20.
Time required: About 1 hour.
Materials and/or environment required: A large, comfortable room and a circle of straight-backed chairs.

Process

1. The facilitator asks the group to divide into pairs.
2. Each pair nominates one of them as 'A' and one as 'B.'
3. 'A' talks to 'B' for 5 minutes about one of the following topics:
    (a) the house/flat that I live in
    (b) my family
    (c) my political beliefs.
4. 'B' listens to 'A' and observes the SOLER behaviours. Thus she:
    (a) sits squarely
    (b) maintains an open position
    (c) leans slightly towards to the other person
    (d) maintains steady and comfortable eye contact
    (e) relaxes.

'B' may also use minimal prompts but uses them sparingly and consciously.

5. After 5 minutes, roles are reversed and 'B' talks to 'A' for 5 minutes whilst 'A' maintains the SOLER behaviours and uses appropriate minimal prompts.
6. When both aspects of the exercise have been completed, the group is reconvened and the facilitator leads a discussion on what happened.

Evaluation

The facilitator may want to ask the group:

- Was this better or worse that the previous exercise?
- What was it like to be listened to?
- What was it like to listen to the other person?

Notes

It is important that the facilitator emphasizes that this is not a conversation. The listeners should restrict themselves to minimal prompts and not respond in any other way to what their partners say.

It is possible to experiment with the exaggerated negative role play, described above. Using this approach, group members are encouraged to try out using the SOLER behaviours in an exaggerated way. It is advised, however, that the negative approach is used sparingly and not as a routine part of interpersonal skills training. In fact it is important that *no* aspects of interpersonal skills training become routine. The secret, here, is continuously to modify your approach. If, as a trainer, you find yourself getting into a rut, it is likely that the people in your groups will be getting into one too.

Exercise 8

Aim of the exercise: To reinforce the skills of listening and attending with appropriate verbal and non-verbal behaviours.
Group size: Any number from 6 to 20.
Time required: About $1-1\frac{1}{2}$ hours.
Materials and/or environment required: A large, comfortable room and a circle of straight-backed chairs.

Process

1. The facilitator asks the group to divide into threes.
2. The threes are invited to nominate 'A', 'B' and 'C'.
3. 'B' talks to 'B' for 5 minutes on any topic.
4. 'B' listens to 'A' and uses the SOLER behaviours and minimal prompts in an appropriate manner.
5. 'C' acts as a process observer and makes notes on 'B''s performance as a listener.
6. After 5 minutes, each trio feeds back to itself in the following order:
   (a) the listener describes his own performance
   (b) the talker describes the listener's behaviour
   (c) the process observer describes the listener's behaviour.

In each case, it is only the listener's performance that is under discussion.

7. After 10 minutes, 'A', 'B' and 'C' exchange roles and the exercise is repeated. The same assessment procedure is used after the repeat.
8. When all participants have been in the roles of listener, talker and process observer, the facilitator invites the group to reconvene and encourages feedback on the activity.

Notes

The trio's feedback procedure is a vital part of the process of this activity and should not be skipped or rushed. It represents the 'reflection' period of the experiential learning cycle described in earlier chapters. The order of the feedback encourages self-evaluation followed by peer evaluation.

Exercise 9

Aim of the exercise: To test the effectiveness of the listening and attending exercises.
Group size: Any number from 6 to 20.
Time required: About 1–1½ hours.
Materials and/or environment required: A large, comfortable room and a circle of straight-backed chairs.

Process

1. The facilitator asks the group to divide into pairs.
2. Each pair nominates one of them as 'A' and one as 'B'.
3. 'A' talks to 'B' for three periods of 3 minutes, on any topic.
4. 'B' listens to 'A' whilst observing the SOLER behaviours and using appropriate minimal prompts.
5. *Between* each 3-minute period, 'B' paraphrases what 'A' has said, to 'A''s satisfaction. The order is made clear in Figure 6.5.
6. After the cycle has been completed, 'A' and 'B' exchange roles and complete stage 5, above.
7. When the entire cycle has been completed, the facilitator reconvenes the group and invites feedback.

Evaluation

The facilitator may find it useful to ask the following questions:

- What problems did you have with paraphrasing?
- Were all the talkers satisfied with the paraphrasing?
- Could you use paraphrasing in counselling?
- If so, when?

Notes

This exercise can also be used with process observers. Such an observer can be allocated to each pair. Feedback in each trio then takes place as follows:

(a) the listener feeds back on her own performance
(b) the talker offers feedback to the listener
(c) the process observer offers the listener feedback.

---

1. A talks to B for 3 minutes.
2. B paraphrases what A has said.
3. A talks for a further 3 minutes.
4. B paraphrases what A has said.
5. A talks to B for a final 3 minutes.
6. B paraphrases what A has said.

Figure 6.5 The order of Exercise 9

Places I have visited.
What I admire in others.
How I feel about myself.
Common problems I experience in the clinical setting.
What I intend to be doing in 5 years time.
What I did before I came into nursing.
My family.
My views about marriage.
My spiritual beliefs (or lack of them).
What I would do if I wasn't a nurse.
My views on recent news events.
How I feel about the 'green' issues.
How I cope with stress.
How I feel about nursing.
Caring for the elderly.
What I was like as a child.
What I would be like if I was a member of the opposite sex.
How other people see me.
How my parents see me.
A period of history that I would like to have lived through.
Things that make me angry.
Things I like about myself.

Figure 6.6 Topics for use in attending and listening exercises

Once again, the only feedback is to the listener as the aim of the exercise is to encourage and develop listening skills. This exercise further enhances self-monitoring, self-assessment and peer evaluation. A form of this exercise was originally used by Carl Rogers (Kirschenbaum, 1979) as a method of developing client-centred counselling skills.

Figure 6.6 offers a range of topics that can be used for any of the attending and listening skills exercises described in this section. Sometimes, however, it is best to either (a) determine the topics according to current areas of debate within the group or (b) allow group members to decide on their own topics. Group members should always be encouraged to *be themselves* in these exercises and not to act out a particular role. This personalizes the learning that takes place and ensures that the exercises develop skills that can transfer back to the clinical setting.

Exercise 10

Aim of the exercise: To explore the group's need to improve their listening skills.
Group size: Any number from 6 to 20.
Time required: About 20–40 minutes, depending on the size of the group.
Materials and/or environment required: A large, comfortable room and a circle of straight-backed chairs.

Process

1. Each person in turn, completes the statement: 'What I need to do to improve my skills as a listener is ...'. Each group member can complete the statement in any way he chooses.
2. When each person has contributed, the facilitator encourages a discussion about improving listening skills.

Evaluation

The facilitator may like to ask the group:

- What did it feel like to wait your turn in this exercise?
- What similarities and differences are there between group members?
- How *will* people improve their listening skills?

Notes

There are various other statements that can be used in place of the one offered above. Examples include:

- Situations in which I find it difficult to listen include ...
- I don't always listen very well because ...
- I would be a better listener if ...
- If I was a better listener I would ...

Counselling interventions

The bases of effective counselling are the skills of listening and giving attention. Second to these comes the need to use effective verbal interventions. A format for understanding the range of useful and therapeutic interventions has been devised by John Heron (Heron, 1989a) and is called Six Category Intervention Analysis.

This conceptual framework was developed by Heron out of the work of Blake and Mouton (1976). It was offered as a conceptual model for understanding interpersonal relationships, and as an assessment tool for identifying a range of possible therapeutic interactions between two people.

The six categories in Heron's analysis are: prescriptive (offering advice), informative (offering information), confronting (challenging), cathartic (enabling the expression of pent-up emotions), catalytic ('drawing out') and supportive (confirming or encouraging) (Figure 6.7). The word 'intervention' is used to describe any statement that the practitioner may use. The word 'category' is used to denote a range of related interventions.

Heron (1989a) calls the first three categories of intervention (prescriptive, informative and confronting) 'authoritative', and suggests that in using these categories the practitioner retains control over the relationship. He calls the second three categories of intervention (cathartic,

Category	What the counsellor/nurse does
Authoritative interventions	
1. Prescriptive	Makes suggestions, recommends behaviours, offers advice.
2. Informative	Gives new knowledge or information.
3. Confronting	Challenges what the other person says or does.
Facilitative interventions	
4. Cathartic	Helps the other person to release pent-up feelings and emotions.
5. Catalytic	Helps to 'draw out' the other person.
6. Supportive	Encourages and affirms the worth of the other person.

Figure 6.7 The six categories of therapeutic intervention (after Heron, 1989a)

catalytic and supportive) 'facilitative', and suggests that these enable the client to retain control over the relationship. In other words, the first three are 'practitioner-centred' and the second three are 'client-centred'. Another way of describing the difference between the first and second sets of three categories is that the first three are 'You tell me' interventions and the second three are 'I tell you' interventions.

What, then, is the value of such an analysis of therapeutic interventions? First, it identifies the *range* of possible interventions available to the nurse/counsellor. Very often, in day-to-day interactions with others, we stick to repetitive forms of conversation and response simply because we are not aware that other options are available to us. This analysis identifies an exhaustive range of types of human interventions. Second, by identifying the sorts of interventions we can use, we can act more precisely and with a greater sense of intention. The nurse–patient relationship thus becomes more particular and less haphazard: we know *what* we are saying and also *how* we are saying it. We have greater interpersonal choice.

Third, the analysis offers an instrument for training. Once the categories have been identified, they can be used for students and others to identify their weaknesses and strengths across the interpersonal spectrum. Nurses can, in this way, develop a wide and comprehensive range of interpersonal skills.

It is worth repeating that the skills identified in this chapter as counselling skills are exactly similar to the basic human skills used in day to day nursing interactions. Thus an understanding of the full range of the six categories can enhance and enrich the quality of the nurse's approach to care. It should be noted, too, that the analysis does not offer a mechanical approach to interpersonal skills training. The exercises here will not simply be a training in learning particular phrases and responses. This is an important issue. The analysis indicates a *type* of response. The choice of words, the tone of voice, the non-verbal aspects of a particular response must develop out of the individual's belief and value system and out of their life experience. Those aspects of the response are also dependent upon the situation at the time and upon the people involved. All human relationships occur within a particular context. It is impossible to identify what will necessarily be the right thing to do in *this* situation at *this* time. A mechanical, learning-by-heart approach to counselling or interpersonal skills would, therefore, be inappropriate. In the descriptions of the following exercises, examples are offered but when the exercises are carried out, each student will have to find his own words, his own expressions and his own personal approach. This affirms the basic principle of human skills training: the honouring of personal experience developed through observation and reflection.

Cultural awareness

While counselling is widely recognized as a reasonable practice in so-called Western countries, it is certainly not the only approach to personal problem-solving. In particular, the client-centred approach to counselling, in which the person receiving counselling is encouraged to identify his or her own problems and also their solutions, is acceptable only in cultures that value individualism and the primacy of the individual. Anyone working in multicultural settings (and that must surely include most nurses) must remain sensitive to cultural differences amongst client groups. While it is beyond the scope of this book to highlight particular cultural issues involved in counselling, it is valuable to note McLeod's (1998) guidelines for multicultural counselling practice. His guidelines were derived from the work of Johnson and Nadirshaw (1993) and Pedersen (1994) and are as follows.

> There is no single concept of 'normal' that applies across all persons, situations and cultures. Mainstream concepts of mental health and illness must be expanded to incorporate religious and spiritual elements. It is important to take a flexible and respectful approach to other therapeutic values, beliefs and traditions: we must each of us assume that our own view is to some extent culturally biased.

> Individualism is not the only way to view human behaviour, and must be supplemented by collectivism in some situations. Dependency is not a bad characteristic in all cultures.

> It is essential to acknowledge the reality of racism and discrimination in the lives of clients, and in the therapy process. Power imbalances between therapists and clients may reflect the imbalance of power between the cultural communities in which they belong.

> Language use is important: abstract 'middle-class' psychotherapeutic discourse may not be understood by people coming from other cultures. Linear thinking/ story telling is not universal.

> It is important to take account of the structures within the client's community that serve to strengthen and support the client: natural supporting methods are important to the individual. For some clients, traditional healing methods may be more effective that Western forms of counselling.

It is necessary to take history into account when making sense of current experience. The way that someone feels may not only be a response to what is happening now, but in part a response to loss or trauma that occurred in earlier generations.

Be willing to talk about cultural and racial issues and differences in the counselling room.

Check it out with the client – be open to learning from the client. (McLeod, 1998)

Almost all of the above points can be adapted to communication in everyday nursing practice. It is easy, perhaps, for all of us to be ethnocentric – to believe that the way we do things is in some way the 'right' way. Only by studying cultures and by listening closely to what clients, patients and colleagues are telling us about other cultures will we begin to avoid this trap.

Nurses' perceptions of their interpersonal skills

We invited both student nurses and trained nursing staff to identify their own strengths and weaknesses in terms of the Six Category Intervention Analysis (Burnard and Morrison, 1988; Morrison and Burnard, 1989). In the first study, using a random sample of 92 trained nurses, those nurses were asked to rank order the six categories according to how skilful they thought they were in using them. Generally speaking the nurses perceived themselves to be more skilled in using the authoritative categories and less skilled in using the facilitative categories. Having said that, *most of the nurses perceived themselves as being particularly weak in using cathartic* and *catalytic* interventions. Overall, they perceived themselves as being best at being supportive.

There were marked similarities in the findings of the second study in which we invited 84 student nurses to rank order the six categories in terms of their perceived strengths and weaknesses in using them. Again we found an overall picture of greater perceived skill in using authoritative interventions rather than facilitative ones. Students also thought that they were generally most effective in using supportive interventions and not so good at using cathartic and confronting interventions. In general, the results of both studies support Heron's (1989a) assertion that a wide range of practitioners in our society show a much greater deficit in the skilful use of facilitative interventions than they do in the skilful use of authoritative ones.

Using the exercises

Two principles would be observed when using the exercises in this section. Participation in them should always be voluntary. Growth in interpersonal development can never be enhanced if participation is enforced. This, then, is the *voluntary principle*. The other principle – as

1. Prescriptive	(a) 'Perhaps you would like to talk to your family about this'.
	(b) 'I suggest you talk to your GP about the rash'.
2. Informative	(a) 'These tablets may make you feel a bit drowsy'.
	(b) 'There is a *Relate* office in . . .'.
3. Confronting	(a) 'We agreed to stop at 3 pm, so we will stop now'.
	(b) 'I notice that you very frequently talk about how much you hate your husband and you also say that you will stay with him . . .'.
4. Cathartic	(a) 'It's all right with me if you want to cry'.
	(b) 'What do you *really* want to say now . . .'.
5. Catalytic	(a) 'Can you say more . . .'.
	(b) 'What happened then?
6. Supportive	(a) 'I appreciate your being here'.
	(b) 'I enjoy spending time with you'.

Figure 6.8   Examples of interventions within the six categories

mentioned in the previous chapter – is the *gymnasium principle* (Heron, 1977b). Just as a gymnast exercises one set of muscles in isolation to the rest that would not normally be used in that way, so the exercises that follow pick out one small aspect of the counselling relationship. Just as the gymnast later feels the benefit of exercising different sets of muscles, so the nurse feels more interpersonally competent when she has undertaken the whole range of activities described here. The learning from particular exercises needs to be incorporated into everyday life just as the gymnast needs to use all his muscles in day-to-day living.

Figure 6.8 offers some examples of interventions within the six categories. It must be repeated, however, that the important issue is that such interventions develop naturally out of the context the nurse and patient find themselves in. The examples are offered only as a means of clarifying the concept of the six categories and not as exemplars or as 'ideal types'.

In a more general sense, the six categories of intervention have a wider application, beyond the counselling relationship. The nurse working in a hospice, for example, may need considerable cathartic skills in order to enable the expression of feelings. The charge nurse will require prescriptive skills when delegating ward duties. All nurses require the ability to be appropriately supportive. Nurse educators will find that the whole range of interventions can be used in the contexts of teaching and learning. Indeed the process of experiential learning is particularly facilitated by the skilful use of the cathartic, catalytic and supportive categories.

There may be situations in which skilful use of a *particular* category may be required in this way. The nurse who is skilled in all six categories can deftly select the appropriate category for the right situation. Figure 6.9 shows some examples of nursing situations in which one particular category can be used. They can *only* be examples. It is acknowledged that the stated category would always be used *along with* others. The examples do,

Prescriptive Interventions	1. When delegating nursing duties. 2. Advising people prior to discharge. 3. Enabling students to develop a conceptual framework.
Informative Interventions	1. During the admission of new patients. 2. Reporting to other health professionals. 3. During teaching sessions.
Confronting Interventions	1. When antisocial behaviour occurs. 2. When incorrect nursing procedures are used. 3. During multidisciplinary meetings.
Cathartic Interventions	1. While counselling relatives. 2. While caring for the spiritually distressed. 3. While caring for the dying.
Catalytic Interventions	1. During clinical teaching sessions. 2. While talking to patients while compiling care plans. 3. While counselling the distressed or uncertain person.
Supportive Interventions	1. During all nursing situations. 2. During all teaching situations. 3. Throughout all human interactions.

Figure 6.9 Examples of nursing situations in which skills of a particular category may be used

however, make concrete, the abstract: they show the practical application of the six category approach in everyday nursing life.

One last point needs to be made here: not *all* the categories will be used in *every* social or therapeutic encounter. As we have noted all along, the point is to be able to skilfully choose the right approach at the right time.

Also, it may not be for nothing that the nurses in our study felt themselves to be most skilled in being supportive. Everyone needs support and encouragement. Everyone needs to be affirmed. Or as Martin Buber put it: 'Man wishes to be confirmed by man ... secretly and bashfully he watches for a Yes which allows him to be and which can only come from one human person to another' (Buber, 1965).

Exercises in using the six categories

The following exercises allow for three phases of personal development:

1. The ability to discriminate between the categories.
2. Ability to use each category skilfully.
3. Applications of the categories to the counselling situation and to the wider nursing context.

Exercise 11

Aim of the exercise: To enhance discrimination between the six categories of therapeutic intervention.
Group size: Any number from 6 to 20.
Time required: Between 40 minutes and 1 hour.
Materials and/or environment required: A large, comfortable room and a circle of straight-backed chairs.

Process

1. The facilitator describes the six categories as outlined above.
2. Group members in turn state a category title and then offer an example of an intervention in that category, e.g. 'Catalytic intervention: "Can you tell me more about what happened?"'.
3. The group decide whether or not the example offered was a true example of an intervention in the stated category.
4. When all group members have offered a category title and an example, a discussion is developed about the use of the analysis.

Evaluation

The facilitator may want to ask:

- What sorts of interventions do you find yourself commonly using?
- What particular interventions do you feel least happy using?

Exercise 12

Aim of the exercise: To enhance discrimination between the six categories.
Group size: Any number from 6 to 20.
Time required: Between 40 minutes and 1 hour.
Materials and/or environment required: A large, comfortable room and a circle of straight-backed chairs.

Process

1. Each group member in turn states, in the first person, something that he may say in a counselling situation. They follow the expression by 'tagging' it with a category label, as per the six categories, e.g. 'It is not possible for you to see the doctor today – informative intervention'.
2. When all group members have offered an expression and a 'tag', a discussion is developed about the use of the analysis.

Evaluation

The facilitator may ask the group:

- How accurate do you feel you are in identifying interventions?
- Were most of the interventions covered in that exercise?

Exercise 13

Aim of the exercise: To enhance discrimination between the six categories.
Group size: Any number from 6 to 20.
Time required: About 1 hour.
Materials and/or environment required: A large, comfortable room and a circle of straight-backed chairs. Notebooks and pens. A white or blackboard.

Process

1. The facilitator reads out each of the following expressions (or writes them on a white or blackboard).
2. Group members are invited to jot down which category each expression fits into.
3. Afterwards, the group discuss their findings.

   The expressions are:

(a) 'What happened when you talked to your wife last night?'
(b) 'How are you feeling at the moment?'
(c) 'I am interested in what you have to say.'
(d) 'The tablets are likely to help the pain.'
(e) 'I suggest you talk to your daughter about this.'
(f) 'I would appreciate it if you stopped doing that'
(g) 'You feel angry at the moment?'
(h) 'I'm very fond of you'.
(i) 'It's OK to cry.'
(j) 'You could enrol on a course at night school.'
(k) 'You are laughing and you say you are angry ...'.
(l) 'Who do I remind you of?'

Evaluation

The facilitator may want to ask:

- What are the problems associated with deciding on a particular category?
- Are there 'good' and 'bad' interventions?

Notes

Some group members are likely to want to know what the 'right' answers are. This can lead to a fruitful debate about personal perceptions and individual choices about what constitutes examples of each category.

Exercise 14

Aim of the exercise: To enhance discrimination between the six categories.
Group size: Any number from 6 to 20.
Time required: About 1 hour.
Materials and/or environment required: A large, comfortable room and a circle of straight-backed chairs. A pack of 24 cards: four marked prescriptive, four marked informative and so on through the categories. The pack should be shuffled.

Process

1. The facilitator passes the pack of cards, face down, to the first group member.
2. The first member picks the first downturned card from the top of the pack and shows it to the group.
3. The group member then offers an example of an intervention from that category.
4. The group decides whether or not the intervention that was offered *was* a true example.
5. When the group is satisfied, the card is placed on the bottom of the pack and the pack is passed to the next group member.
6. Stages 2–5 above are repeated.
7. When all members have completed the round, the facilitator leads a discussion on the outcome.

Exercise 15

Aim of the exercise: To identify individuals' and groups' strengths and deficiencies in the six categories.
Group size: Any number from 6 to 20.
Time required: About 20–30 minutes.
Materials and/or environment required: A large, comfortable room and a circle of straight-backed chairs. A handout, laid out as shown in Figure 6.10, is required for each group member. A flipchart, chalkboard or whiteboard is required, on which is drawn the grid illustrated in Figure 6.11.

Process

1. The facilitator gives each member a handout laid out as shown in Figure 6.10.
2. Each group member ticks the two categories that she feels she currently uses MOST skilfully and puts crosses against the two that she feels she uses LEAST skillfully.
3. When the handouts have been completed, the facilitator collates the results of the assessment on to the grid shown in Figure 6.11.
4. When the group reconvenes, a discussion is held on the outcomes.

Six category intervention analysis skills assessment

Please place a tick beside the *two* categories that you feel you
currently use most skilfully, in any context. Place a cross
beside the *two* categories that you feel you use *least* skilfully
in any context.

	Most skilled	Least skilled
1. Prescriptive		
2. Informative		
3. Confronting		
4. Cathartic		
5. Catalytic		
6. Supportive		

Figure 6.10 Six category intervention analysis skills assessment form

	✓	✗
1. Prescriptive		
2. Informative		
3. Confronting		
4. Cathartic		
5. Catalytic		
6. Supportive		

Figure 6.11 Six category intervention analysis skills assessment grid

Evaluation

The facilitator may want to ask:

- How easy/difficult was this exercise to do?
- Does the ease with which you can use certain interventions depend on the *context*?
- Where you surprised by the outcome of this activity?

Notes

This is a very useful exercise to use at the beginning of a counselling skills
workshop, once group members have grasped the essentials of the six
category approach. Out of the collated results can be decided a format
for concentrating on the development of particular categories that are

identified as areas of weakness. Thus the activity becomes an aspect of the negotiated curriculum. It was this activity that gave us the idea to do the research into nurses' perceptions of their own interpersonal skills (Burnard and Morrison, 1988; Morrison and Burnard, 1989), although different types of ranking and rating scales were used.

Exercises to develop skills in specific categories

Prescriptive skills

Prescriptive interventions involve giving advice, being critical, making suggestions and generally attempting to direct the behaviour of the other person. It is important that prescriptive interventions are made in the true interest of the other person. They should not degenerate into 'putting people's lives right' or into foisting your own set of values onto someone else. Nor should they patronize or oppress.

As a general rule, prescriptive interventions are probably best used to help with concrete life-problems. In other words, it is possible to give advice about, say, moving house or coping with diabetes: it is not so easy to give advice about how another person should live his life.

Exercise 16

Aim of the exercise: To explore the use of prescriptive interventions.
Group size: Any number from 6 to 20.
Time required: About $1\frac{1}{2}$ hours.
Materials and/or environment required: A large, comfortable room and a circle of straight-backed chairs. A flipchart pad, chalkboard or white-board.

Process

1. The facilitator displays the following list of situations.
2. Group members are invited to suggest whether or not they feel that a prescriptive approach would be suitable in helping with those situations.
3. After all of the items have been worked through, the facilitator leads a discussion on the problems of being prescriptive.

The situations are:

(a)   A young patient asks you about how to cope with his colostomy.
(b)   A student nurse wants to know how to cope with the fact that her boyfriend has left her.
(c)   A staff nurse asks you what her next career move should be.
(d)   A patient in a psychiatric unit asks you why he has been prescribed orphenadrine and whether or not he should continue to take it.
(e)   An elderly person asks you what she can do about the fact that he has lost his religious beliefs.
(f)   A young girl asks you for your views on abortion.

Evaluation

The facilitator may want to ask the following questions:

- Can you identify when prescriptive interventions may be appropriate?
- What makes a 'good' prescriptive intervention?

Notes

Giving another person advice is a notoriously difficult thing to do. It is sometimes helpful if the phrase 'Can I make a suggestion ...?' precedes the advice. In this way (at least, in theory!), the other person can choose to listen to or avoid the advice.

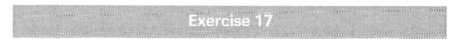

Exercise 17

Aim of the exercise: To develop the use of prescriptive interventions.
Group size: Any number from 6 to 20.
Time required: Between 1 and 2 hours.
Materials and/or environment required: A large, comfortable room and a circle of straight-backed chairs.

Process

1. The facilitator invites the group to sit in silence for 2 minutes and to recall an incident from their lives in which they were given advice.
2. The group is then asked to divide into pairs.
3. Each pair nominates one of them as 'A' and the other as 'B'.
4. 'A' describes the incident to 'B' and 'B' listens without responding in any way.
5. After 5 minutes the facilitator asks 'A' to reflect upon the following questions:
   (a) How well was the advice given?
   (b) Was the advice appropriate?
   (c) How would *you* have delivered such advice?
   (d) Did you *take* the advice?
6. 'A' then ponders on these questions, aloud, in the presence of 'B'.
7. After 5 minutes, the facilitator asks the pair to exchange roles.
8. 'B' then relates his incident to 'A' and ponders on the above questions.
9. When the cycle has been completed, the facilitator invites the group to reconvene.
10. The group identifies the factors that contribute to the legitimate use of prescriptive interventions.

Evaluation

Questions similar to those outlined for the previous exercise can be used here.

Notes

The philosopher Jean-Paul Sartre maintained that we tend to ask advice from those people whose advice we could anticipate (Sartre, 1973). In the end, we have to decide for ourselves.

Exercise 18

Aim of the exercise: To identify valid prescriptive interventions.
Group size: Any number from 6 to 20.
Time required: About 1 hour.
Materials and/or environment required: A large, comfortable room and a circle of straight-backed chairs.

Process

1. The facilitator invites each group member to offer an example of a prescriptive intervention, stated supportively and therapeutically.
2. After each intervention, the group decides:
   (a) Was the intervention an example of a prescriptive intervention?
   (b) Was the manner in which the intervention was offered appropriate?
3. When all group members have offered an intervention, the facilitator convenes a discussion on the therapeutic use of prescriptive interventions.

Notes

This type of exercise is easily modified for *any* of the six categories and is useful for helping to 'cement' the concept of a particular intervention in people's minds.

Informative skills

Informative interventions involve instructing, informing and generally imparting information to the other person. In counselling (and probably in most other situations), informative interventions are probably restricted to factual information and, as with prescriptive interventions, should not be about 'putting people's lives right'.

There has been increasing emphasis placed on information-giving in nursing (Hayward, 1975; Boore, 1978; Devine and Cook, 1983; Engstrom, 1984) and it may be that nurses expect that an important part of their role is giving information to others. This seems quite reasonable when such information is concerned with things like medicine, surgery and other 'factual' situations. It is of less certain value in areas where people are suffering from emotional and personal problems. Whatever the rights and wrongs of giving information, it is undeniable that information when it is given needs to be given clearly, unambiguously and supportively.

Exercise 19

Aim of the exercise: To develop the use of informative interventions.
Group size: Any number from 6 to 20.
Time required: About 1 to 2 hours.
Materials and/or environment required: A large, comfortable room and a circle of straight-backed chairs. Flipchart sheets and large felt-tipped pens.

Process

1. The facilitator divides the group into small sub-groups of three to four people.
2. Each person is asked to recall, silently, two people from their lives:
   (a) one who gave information badly
   (b) one who gave information skilfully.

Examples may be drawn from parents, teachers, lecturers, friends and so forth.

3. In the small groups, group members identify on a flipchart sheet two lists of items:
   (a) the specific behaviours and qualities of the people who gave information badly
   (b) the specific behaviours and qualities of the people who gave information skilfully.
4. After 15 minutes, the group is invited to reconvene and share their findings.
5. The facilitator helps to draw out the necessary behaviours and qualities of the person who gave information skilfully and therapeutically.

Evaluation

The facilitator may want to ask the following questions:

- How effective are YOU at giving information?
- What are the most difficult things about giving information?
- What *sort* of information is difficult to give?

Notes

It is important that all group members are encouraged to practise their listening skills whilst doing these pairs exercises. A useful reminder is to every so often invite the pairs to 'freeze' at the end of an exercise and to notice the position that they and their partner is sitting in. This position can then be compared and contrasted with the SOLER behaviours described above.

Confronting skills

Confronting interventions involve being challenging or giving direct feedback to the other person about their behaviour, attitude and so forth. A

- Direct feedback on behaviour, use of language, attitudes etc.
- Direct feedback on the effects of the other person's behaviour on self and others.
- Challenging illogicalities and inconsistencies.
- Challenging incongruities between what is said and the 'body language' that accompanies it.
- Challenging unaware, unconcious behaviour.
- Drawing attention to contractual behaviour.
- Drawing attention to rules or codes of conduct.

Figure 6.12   Examples of issues for confrontation

confronting intervention challenges the restrictive attitudes, beliefs and behaviours of the other person. Examples of issues on which people may be confronted are identified in Figure 6.12.

Confronting interventions should always be offered supportively and they should never degenerate into an attack on the other person.

Creative confrontation is a struggle between persons who are engaged in a dispute or controversy and who remain together, face to face, until acceptance, respect for differences and love emerge; even though the persons may be at odds with the issue, they are no longer at odds with each other (Moustakas, 1984).

Because the prospect of confronting another person often causes anxiety (for we risk being rebuffed, disagreed with or challenged ourselves), the temptation is either to:

(a)   become aggressive and turn the confrontation into an attack. This is what Heron (1989a) calls the 'sledgehammer' approach; or

(b)   'Pussyfoot', or timidly approach the topic without being clear what the confrontation is really about. The pussyfooter goes all round the houses in a usually vain attempt to avoid saying what she really means.

Figure 6.13 shows a possible range of interventions from the sledge-hammer through to the pussyfoot and identifies confrontation as the centre point. Using confrontation well takes practice. The nature of the nursing profession is such that nurses often feel unable to assert themselves and confront 'cleanly'. As a result, the outcome is often that they either attack or avoid. Our research suggested that confrontation is the skill that some nurses find the most difficult of all the six in this analysis (Burnard and Morrison, 1988; Morrison and Burnard, 1989). Assertiveness training can help here (Bond, 1986) and courses in assertion training are frequently offered by colleges and extra-mural departments of universities. They can be a useful way of developing confronting skills and of furthering self-awareness.

Exercise 20

Aim of the exercise: To practise the use of confronting interventions.
Group size: Any number from 6 to 20.

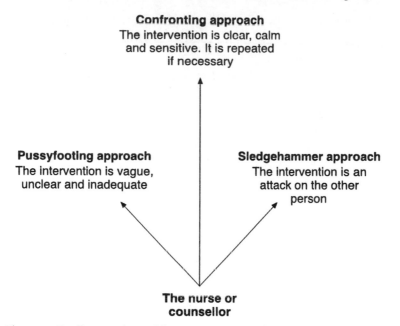

Confronting approach
The intervention is clear, calm
and sensitive. It is repeated
if necessary

Pussyfooting approach
The intervention is vague,
unclear and inadequate

Sledgehammer approach
The intervention is an
attack on the other
person

**The nurse or
counsellor**

Figure 6.13 Range of possible interventions either side of confrontation

Time required: About 2 hours.
Materials and/or environment required: A large, comfortable room and a circle of straight-backed chairs.

Process

1. The facilitator explains that this exercise involves role play and invites the group to break up into sub-groups and decide upon:
   (a) two 'characters'
   (b) one or two process observers.
2. When the sub groups have assembled the following instructions are given:
   (a) One character is a student nurse.
   (b) One character is a charge nurse.
   (c) The student nurse has been reported to the charge nurse regarding *one* of the following issues:
       (i) he or she is persistently late
       (ii) he or she has made sexual advances towards another member of staff
       (iii) he or she has been abusive towards a number of patients.
   (d) The charge nurse's task is to meet the student and to confront him/her on the issue. The charge nurse should be clear, calm and supportive and avoid either the pussyfooting or the sledgehammer approaches.
   (e) The process observer's task is to observe the role play unfolding and to rate the charge nurse on her ability to be skilfully confronting.
3. After the role play has run for 15 minutes, the facilitator invites each sub-group to evaluate their experience in the following manner:
   (a) The charge nurse self-evaluates her performance.
   (b) The student nurse evaluates the charge nurse's performance.

(c) The process observers offer their observations to the charge nurse.

It is important that only the charge nurse's performance is under review. However effective the person was playing the student nurse, the aim is to concentrate on effective confrontation, not on the quality of the acting!

4. When the whole cycle of events has been completed, the facilitator reconvenes the larger group and invites feedback from the sub-groups.
5. Following the plenary session, the group collectively identify what behaviours and qualities make for successful confrontation.

Evaluation

The facilitator may want to ask:

- What are *you* like at confrontation?
- What are the specific problems involved in confronting another person?
- *Who* do you confront best?
- Who would you *least like* to confront?

Notes

As this is role play, it is important that the people who have been role playing are de-briefed after the exercise. This may be achieved by each actor disassociating from the role by describing to the group one of the following:

(a)   A recent pleasant experience.
(b)   Interests away from the group and away from work.
(c)   Their job in real life.

This exercise can be adapted to suit the particular nursing group taking part. More difficult topics can be chosen for more senior staff. Groups may also be invited to choose their own topics for role play.

The technical details of trade union representation and the grievance procedure do not normally go unquestioned during this activity and can serve as useful material for discussion!

Cathartic skills

Being human is a complicated business. It is complicated further by our emotional make-up. We experience joy and pain, laugher and disappointment. We also all have a tendency to bottle up emotion. Cathartic interventions are those that help the other person to explore their feelings and, as necessary, to express them, through laughter, anger, trembling or tears. We live in a culture where the free expression of feelings is not the norm. Given that they are often helping people who are likely to be emotional, it is important that nurses learn skills in helping in this domain.

Types of emotion

John Heron (1977) distinguishes between at least four types of emotion that are frequently suppressed or bottled up: anger, fear, grief and embarrassment. He suggests a relationship between these feelings and certain overt expressions of them. Thus, anger may be expressed as loud sound, fear as trembling, grief through tears and embarrassment through laughter. He notes, also, a relationship between those feelings and certain basic human needs. Firstly, Heron argues that we all have the need to understand and know what is happening to us. If that knowledge is not forthcoming, we may experience fear. Secondly, we need to make choices in our lives and if that choice is restricted in certain ways, we may feel anger. Thirdly, we need to experience the expression of love and of being loved. If that love is not forthcoming or if it is taken away from us, we experience grief. Finally, to Heron's basic human needs may be added the need for self respect and dignity. If such dignity is denied us, we may feel self-conscious and embarrassed. Figure 6.14 illustrates some of the effects of bottling up emotion over a long period.

Coping with other people's emotions

Different people react in different ways to the bottling up of emotion in the same way. Some people, too, choose not to deal with life events emotionally. It would be odd to argue that there is a 'norm' where emotions are concerned. On the other hand, many people complain of being unable to cope with emotions and if the person being counselled perceives there to be a problem in the emotional domain, then that perception may be expressed as a desire to explore her emotional status. It is important, however, that the nurse does not force his particular set of beliefs about feelings and emotions on to the other person, but waits to be asked to help. There should be no question that we force cathartic counselling on others under the belief we may have that emotional release is 'good for you'. Sometimes it is: sometimes it isn't.

Drawing on the literature on the subject, the following statements may be made about the handling of emotions:

- Emotional release is usually self-limiting. If the person is allowed to cry or get angry, that emotion will be expressed and then gradually subside.
- There seems to be a link between the amount we can 'allow' another person to express emotion and the degree to which we can handle our own emotion. This

---

- Physical discomfort and muscular pain; particularly muscular discomfort.
- Difficulty in decision making.
- Problems with self-image.
- Difficulty in setting realistic goals.
- The development of long-term faulty beliefs.
- The 'last straw' syndrome; lashing out at objects or at other people.

Figure 6.14 Some effects of bottling up emotion

is another reason why nurses need self-awareness. To help others explore their feelings we need, first, to explore our own.

- Touch can often be helpful in the form of holding the person's hand or putting an arm round them. Care should be taken, however, that such actions are unambiguous: for some, touch always has sexual connotations. It is worth remembering, too, that not everyone likes or wants physical contact. It is important the nurse's support is not intrusive.
- Once a person has had an emotional release she will need time to piece together the insights gained from such release. Often all that is needed is that the nurse sits quietly with the other person while she occasionally verbalizes what she is thinking. The post cathartic period can be a very important stage in the cathartic process.
- Certain counselling interventions can help in the exploration of feelings and in the promotion of emotional release. These are illustrated in Figure 6.15.

There are a number of ways in which the nurse can develop skills in exploring and expressing emotions in themselves and in others. Co-counselling offers a simple and effective means of gaining cathartic competence (Bond, 1986) Gestalt therapy workshops also help in the process of handling feelings. Both methods are frequently taught in short courses run by colleges and extramural departments of universities.

The examples shown in Figure 6.15 are but a few of many methods of helping in the expression of emotion. All of them, used deftly and skilfully can enable the client to explore her emotions. All of them, too are also

Type of cathartic intervention	Example
1. Giving permission	'It's all right with me if you cry . . .'.
2. Helping remove physical blocks	'Try taking three deep breaths . . . open your eyes really wide . . .'.
3. Picking up on sudden physical gestures	'Try exaggerating that arm movement . . . that facial expression . . .'.
4. Noting mismatches between verbal and non-verbal behaviours	'You say you're upset and you're smiling'.
5. Inviting repitition of emotionally charged statements, offered by the client	'Try saying 'I'm angry', again . . . and again . . .'.
6. Exploring fantasy	'If you could do whatever you wanted, what would you do?'
7. Mobilization of body energy	'Stand up and stretch . . . shake yourself vigorously.'
8. Literal description of a place that the client has talked about	'You talked about your old house . . . describe one of the rooms to me . . . in detail.'
9. Exploring hidden agendas	'Who are you *really* saying that too?'
10. Role-playing relationships	'If your mother was here now, what would you say to her? What has been left unsaid?
11. Catching fleeting thoughts	'Noting fleeting eye movements and asking: 'What are you thinking? . . . What's the thought?'

Figure 6.15   Examples of cathartic interventions

useful 'alternative' counselling techniques for helping to liberate new trains of thought, fresh solutions and different perspectives on distressing issues. It is suggested that their use be explored gently and carefully in training workshops and that nurses become skilled in using them *with each other* before they begin to use them in the clinical situation. It is also recommended that facilitators who work a lot in the cathartic domain should first receive training in cathartic methods.

Exercise 21

Aim of the exercise: To explore emotional areas in group members' experience.
Group size: Any number from 6 to 20.
Time required: Between 1 and $1\frac{1}{2}$ hours.
Materials and/or environment required: A large, comfortable room and a circle of straight-backed chairs.

Process

1. The facilitator explains that the aim of the exercise is to explore emotion and that expression of emotion during the exercise is quite acceptable.
2. The facilitator invites the group to divide into pairs.
3. Each pair nominates one of them as 'A' and one as 'B'.
4. 'A' talks to 'B', uninterrupted on one of the following topics:
   (a) early childhood experiences
   (b) my relationship with my family
   (c) what I would tell you about myself if I knew you really well
   (d) what I worry about most of all
   (e) what makes me happy and unhappy.
5. 'B' gives 'A' attention only and does not interrupt.
6. After 10 minutes, 'A' and 'B' exchange roles and work through the exercise again.
7. After all group members have completed the cycle, the group reconvenes and discusses the experience. There should, however, be no discussion of the CONTENT of the pairs' work. That should remain confidential to the pairs concerned. Instead, the discussion should focus on what the *feelings* generated.
8. At the end of the allotted time, the facilitator invites each member of the group to describe something that he or she is looking forward to. This serves to 'lighten' the atmosphere and to end the session on a positive note.

Evaluation

The facilitator may like to ask:

- What sorts of *feelings* emerged?
- What did you *do* with those feelings?
- How do you normally cope with your own feelings?
- What do you do when other people express emotion?

Exercise 22

Aim of the exercise: To practise the use of cathartic interventions.
Group size: Any number from 6 to 20.
Time required: Between 1 and $1\frac{1}{2}$ hours.
Materials and/or environment required: A large, comfortable room and a circle of straight-backed chairs.

Process

1. The facilitator outlines a variety of cathartic interventions and demonstrates their use.
2. The group divides into pairs.
3. Each pair nominates one of them as 'A' and the other as 'B'.
4. 'A' talks to 'B' and 'B' uses a limited number of cathartic interventions from the list above. Only cathartic interventions are used. Suitable topics for the exercise are:
   (a) my feelings about my life so far
   (b) my feelings about my family
   (c) my relationships with close friends
   (d) my relationship with myself.
5. After 10 minutes, the pairs swap roles.
6. When all group members have completed the cycle of events, the facilitator reconvenes the group and invites a discussion on the experiences of group members. Again, the CONTENT of what was talked about is not discussed. The focus of the discussion should be:
   (a) the feelings of group members
   (b) the ease or difficulty of using cathartic interventions.

Notes

It is sometimes helpful if a video tape can be prepared and shown to the group on the skilled use of cathartic interventions. Alternatively, the facilitator can demonstrate their use with a skilled person brought into the group for the purpose.

Catalytic skills

> When you ask me how I feel, I'm the only one who can tell you! And I like that!
>
> (Primary school child quoted by Canfield and Wells, 1976)

Catalytic interventions are those that involve drawing the person out through the use of open questions, reflection and empathy building. Examples of such interventions are illustrated in Figure 6.16. Of all of these, questions, perhaps, are the most frequently used of all interpersonal interventions. Hargie, Saunders and Dickson (1994) suggest that the general functions of questions are as follows:

Open questions:
An open question is one that has potential for the client to develop. It does not require a 'yes' or a 'no' answer.
e.g. 'How do you feel about what's happening at home?'
Open questions tend to begin with: 'How', 'What', 'When' or 'Why'.

Reflection
Reflection is the technique of repeating or paraphrasing the last few words of the other person's utterance, e.g.
Client: 'I left home and found life very difficult. I couldn't settle and didn't know what I should do . . .'.
Nurse: 'You weren't sure what to do . . .'.
It is helpful if 'reflections' do not become 'questions', through the nurse's tone of voice and inflection. The 'reflection' should be a 'mirror' image of the last few words spoken by the other person.

Empathy building
Empathy building involves the nurse intuitively assessing the feeling of the other person and verbalizing that assessment, e.g.
'You sound very angry'.
'That must have been very upsetting . . .'.

Figure 6.16 Examples of catalytic interventions

to obtain information;
to maintain control of the interaction;
to arouse interest and curiosity;
to diagnose specific difficulties a respondent may have;
to express an interest in the respondent;
to ascertain the attitudes, feelings and opinions of the respondent;
to encourage maximum participation by the respondent;
to assess the extent of the respondent's knowledge;
to encourage critical thought and evaluation;
to communicate, in group discussions, that involvement and overt participation by all group members is expected and valued;
to encourage group members to comment on the responses of other members of the group;
to maintain the attention of group members, by asking questions, periodically, without advance warning.

Exercise 23

Aim of the exercise: To discriminate between open and closed questions.
Group size: Any number from 6 to 20.
Time required: Between 40 minutes and 1 hour.
Materials and/or environment required: A large, comfortable room and a circle of straight-backed chairs. Handouts marked O.C.C.O.O.C.

Process

1. The facilitator demonstrates the difference between open and closed questions.
2. The group divides into pairs.
3. Each pair nominates one of them as 'A' and one as 'B'.
4. 'A' then asks questions of 'B' in the order on the handouts (open, closed, closed, open, open, closed). Suitable topics for this exercise include:
   (a) the River Thames
   (b) veteran cars
   (c) steel tubes
   (d) favourite pictures

These topics are useful because they elicit short answers and thus keep the exercise brisk. If emotive or interesting (!) topics are used, the exercise is likely to take a long time and the point of sticking to open and closed questions may be lost.

5. At the end of the first cycle of questions, the pairs exchange roles and the other person works through the list of questions.
6. When all group members have asked the series of questions and have been asked questions, the facilitator invokes a discussion on the process of asking questions.

Evaluation

The facilitator may like to ask:

- When would you use open questions in preference to closed questions?
- When would closed questions be appropriate?
- What sort of questions do you ask most frequently in the clinical situation?

Exercise 24

Aim of the exercise: To explore the use of 'why' questions.
Group size: Any number from 6 to 20.
Time required: Between 1 and 2 hours.
Materials and/or environment required: A large, comfortable room and a circle of straight-backed chairs.

Process

1. The facilitator invites the group to break into pairs.
2. Each of the pairs nominates one of them as 'A' and one as 'B'.
3. 'A' then talks to 'B' about his or her effectiveness as a counsellor.
4. As the conversation unfolds, 'B' asks a continuous series of 'why' questions of 'A'. Thus the conversation may sound a bit like this:
   A: I am fairly good at talking to relatives ... except when they start getting emotional ...
   B: Why do you find it difficult when they get emotional?
   A: Because it makes *me* emotional, I suppose.

B: Why does it make you feel emotional?
A: It reminds me of my own problems ...
B: Why does it do that?

And so on.

5. The pair continue in this way for 10 minutes. and then exchange roles. 'A' asks 'why' questions of 'B'.
6. When the exercise has been completed, the group re-forms and the facilitator leads a discussion on what happened.

Evaluation

It is useful to consider the following questions:

- How did it feel to be asked a series of 'why' questions?
- What are the good and bad points about 'why' questions?
- How can 'why' questions be used in counselling?
- When are they best avoided?

Notes

This activity was developed out of Hinckle's 'laddering' process: a research method used to explore belief and value systems. It is described in greater detail by Bannister and Fransella (1986). The activity also explores the problems associated with asking 'Why?' questions in counselling.

Exercise 25

Aim of the exercise: To experience being asked a wide range of questions.
Group size: Any number from 6 to 20.
Time required: Between 1 and $1\frac{1}{2}$ hours.
Materials and/or environment required: A large, comfortable room and a circle of straight-backed chairs.

Process

1. The facilitator invites the group to divide into pairs.
2. Each pair nominates one of them as 'A' and one as 'B'.
3. 'A' asks 'B' questions on *any topic at all*, continuously.
4. 'B' *does not answer* any of the questions but merely experiences the feelings that go with being asked them.
5. After 10 minutes 'A' and 'B' exchange roles.
6. When all the group members have completed the cycle, the group facilitator invites the group to reconvene and to discuss the experience.

Evaluation

The facilitator may want to ask:

- What did it feel like *not* to answer questions?
- Did anyone break the rule?
- Did you answer the questions 'silently'?
- What is it like to be bombarded with questions?

Notes

This can be a powerful exercise for demonstrating how intrusive some forms of questioning can be. The facilitator may want to suggest that the group members ask some 'risky' questions – reminding them that at no time are *answers* required!

Exercise 26

Aim of the exercise: To develop the use of reflection.
Group size: Any number from 6 to 20.
Time required: Between 40 minutes and 1 hour.
Materials and/or environment required: A large, comfortable room and a circle of straight-backed chairs.

Process

1. The facilitator describes and demonstrates the technique of reflection.
2. The facilitator asks the group to divide into pairs.
3. Each pair is nominated 'A' and 'B'.
4. 'A' talks to 'B' and 'B' reflects appropriately. Reflection is the only intervention used. Any topic may be chosen for this activity.
5. After 10 minutes, 'A' and 'B' exchange roles and repeat the process.
6. When all group members have worked through the cycle, the facilitator invites the group to reconvene and encourages discussion of the difficulties and value of reflection.

Evaluation

The facilitator may want to ask:

- When would you use reflection?
- When would you avoid it?

Notes

It is interesting to show a video tape of a television interview as an example of the effective use of reflection. Alternatively, the facilitator may ask a colleague to come into the room and demonstrate effective reflection with the facilitator. Reflection is one of the most important forms of communication in counselling. Drawing from the work of a range of other writers, Hargie, Saunders and Dickson (1994) – writing from the point of view of the interviewer – identify the following functions of reflection and these can be useful as a point of discussion in interpersonal skills training:

To demonstrate an interest in and involvement with the interviewee.

To indicate close attention by the interviewer to what is being communicated.

To show that the interviewer is trying to understand fully the interviewee and what the latter is saying.

To check the interviewer's perceptions and ensure accuracy of understanding.

To facilitate the interviewee's comprehension of the issues involved and clarity of thinking on those matters.

To focus attention upon particular aspects and encourage further exploration.

To communicate a deep concern for that which the interviewee considers to be important.

To place the major emphasis upon the interviewee rather than the interviewer in the interviewing situation.

To indicate that it is acceptable for the interviewee to have and express feelings in this situation and to facilitate their ventilation.

To help the interviewee to 'own' feelings.

To enable the interviewee to realize that feelings can be an important cause of behaviour.

To help the interviewee to scrutinize underlying reasons and motives.

To demonstrate the interviewer's ability to empathize with the interviewee.

Exercise 27

Aim of the exercise: To develop a range of catalytic interventions.
Group size: Any number from 6 to 20.
Time required: Between 1 and $1\frac{1}{2}$ hours.
Materials and/or environment required: A large, comfortable room and a circle of straight-backed chairs.

Process

1. The facilitator asks the group to divide into pairs.
2. Each pair nominates one of them as 'A' and one as 'B'.
3. 'A' talks to 'B' using ONLY the following sorts of interventions:
   (a) open questions
   (b) reflections
   (c) empathy building statements.

Thus 'A' initiates the conversation with 'B'.

4. After 10 minutes the facilitator invites the pairs to exchange roles.
5. When all group members have completed the cycle, the facilitator encourages a discussion on their experiences.

Evaluation

The facilitator may want to ask:

- Which sorts of interventions were most difficult to use?
- Which were easiest to use?

Notes

A useful variation on this exercise is to invite the pairs to use the catalytic interventions as clumsily as possible. As we noted previously, 'doing it wrong' can often be a powerful training tool.

This exercise is the first one in which 'A' *initiates* a conversation. It is a useful activity for enabling nurses to consider how to start a conversation with a patient, relative or colleague.

Supportive skills

Supportive interventions are those that involve approving, confirming or validating the other person's experience. The interventions should be genuine, appropriate and never patronizing, paternal or maternal. Neither should they be used 'automatically' as positive reinforcement. It is notable that some nurses are compulsive carers and may *overuse* the supportive category. Overuse of support encourages dependence and disallows the other person from learning from their own experience through standing on their own feet.

Exercise 28

Aim of the exercise: To develop the use of supportive interventions.
Group size: Any number from 6 to 20.
Time required: Between 1 and $1\frac{1}{2}$ hours.
Materials and/or environment required: A large, comfortable room and a circle of straight-backed chairs.

Process

1. Each group member receives validation from each other member of the group. In order to facilitate this, the sentence 'The qualities I like most about you are ...' may be used. The validatory comments should be genuine and un-qualified. Look out for statements that have a 'but' in them!
2. When each member of the group has received validation from every other member, the facilitator invites discussion on the experience.

Evaluation

The facilitator may want to ask:

- What did it feel like to be validated in this way?
- Where there any surprises?
- Did you enjoy the process?
- How effective are you at telling patients and other colleagues that you like them?

Aim of the exercise: To explore self-validation.
Group size: Any number from 6 to 20.
Time required: About 1 hour.
Materials and/or environment required: A large, comfortable room and a circle of straight-backed chairs.

Process

1. Each member of the group, in turn, identifies three or four of their *own* positive characteristics or qualities, to the group.
2. When each person has spoken in this way, the facilitator leads a discussion on self-perception.

Evaluation

The facilitator may want to ask:

- What were other people's views of the qualities chosen by individuals?
- Does anyone want to *add* qualities to the lists that people offered?

Conclusion

When individual categories of interventions have been developed, the group may take longer periods in the pairs format attempting to use the whole range of categories. Alternatively, group exercises may be used such as the ones for discriminating between the categories as described at the beginning of this section.

Once the exercises have been experienced, a commitment must be made by each group member to practise the use of the interventions in the clinical situation. The exercises are of little value if the learning from them stays within the group or within the room. It is vital that the interventions become incorporated into the person's personal style. Once this is the case, the need to notice what interventions we are using becomes less necessary: the interventions have become the person. Sometimes the transitional phase between first learning to discriminate between the six categories and successfully incorporating them into self-presentation is experienced as a period of clumsiness and self-consciousness. Any new learning and any new skills development must cause change in the sense of self and such a period normal passes into one of development of a natural, spontaneous sense of self which is broadened and deepened by the wider choice that the analysis offers.

What has been argued and developed in this chapter is that the skilled nurse has self-awareness. She can *choose* the interventions that she uses and use them both skilfully and appropriately. Such a skilled person has both listening and attending skills. She also has skills in making suggestions, giving information, challenging, drawing out, helping to release emotion and supporting. All of these skills need to be practised in an atmosphere of concern for and appreciation of the worth of the other person. The development of these human skills through personal experience will enhance and enrich the nurse's approach to patient care.

These are the skills and qualities of the one-to-one relationship. In the next chapter, the group process is examined and exercises in developing group skills are explored. Finally, in this chapter, a programme for using the attending, listening and counselling skills exercises is offered as a framework for planning a workshop or course.

A programme for counselling skills training

Introductions

1. The group facilitator introduces the aims of the workshop and outlines domestic arrangements: meal breaks and tea and coffee breaks.
2. The facilitator invites the group members to introduce themselves using the approach outlined in this book. Icebreakers can also be used as required.
3. The facilitator discusses the aims of the workshop and introduces the two principles:
   (a) The voluntary principle: that everyone is free to take part in activities or to sit out of them as they see fit.
   (b) The proposal clause: that group members should take responsibility for suggesting that the group either spends more time on a certain section of the workshop or that things are speeded up.

Theory input

1. The facilitator offers a short theory input on the principles of counselling, including:
   (a) definitions of counselling
   (b) qualities of an effective counselling
   (c) how counselling fits into nursing practice
   (d) the facilitator makes a distinction between two aspects of counselling skills
   (e) attending and listening
   (f) counselling interventions.
2. Experiential learning activities:
   (a) The group then concentrates on attending and listening skills and work through a series of exercises (e.g. Exercises Nos. 1–10 from this book).
   (b) After a plenary session to discuss all aspects of attending and listening, the facilitator moves the group on to counselling interventions.
   (c) The concept of Six Category Intervention Analysis is introduced and dis-

cussed and group members assess their own skills in terms of the six through using the assessment sheet outlined on p. 186.
(d) Out of that assessment, a group profile is drawn up using the grid on p. 187.
(e) The group then concentrate on the three categories that are generally perceived as those requiring most attention.
(f) The group work through a series of exercises to develop skills in the six categories (e.g. a selection from Exercises 11–29 from this book).
(g) Group members are encouraged to work in pairs for longer periods (between 30 minutes and 1 hour as 'A' or 'B') to reinforce the skills learned.

Evaluation and application

1. A final plenary session is held to discuss the application of the new skills to the clinical or community setting.
2. The facilitator leads a evaluation session and closes the workshop.

This format can be adapted for use as a 1- or 2-day workshop, a week-long workshop or as a series of study days.

Recommended reading

Bond, T. (2000) *Standards and Ethics for Counselling in Action*, 2nd edn. London, Sage.
Bor, R. and McCann, D. (eds) (1999) *The Practice of Counselling in Primary Care*. London, Sage.
Feltham, C. (ed.) (1999) *Understanding the Counselling Relationship*. London, Sage.
Holloway, E. and Carroll, M. (eds) (1999) *Training Counselling Supervisors: Strategies, Methods and Techniques*. London, Sage.
Lapworth, P., Sills, C. and Fish, S. (2001) *Integration in Counselling and Psychotherapy: Developing a Personal Approach*. London, Sage.
McLeod, J. (1999) *Practitioner Research in Counselling*. London, Sage.
Mearnes, D. and Thorne, B. (1999) *Person-Centred Counselling in Action*, 2nd edn. London, Sage.
Nelson-Jones, R. (1999) *Introduction to Counselling Skills: Text and Activities*. London, Sage.

7

Experiential Exercises for Human Skills: 2 Group Skills

We all live and work in a variety of types of groups. If the counselling process as outlined and discussed in the previous chapter is comparable to any one-to-one encounter, similarly the group process mirrors any situation in nursing in which three or more people meet. In the nursing profession the individual joins many groups: the training and educational group in the school of nursing, the nursing team on the ward, a variety of meetings, case conferences and so forth. Figure 7.1 identifies some of the many groups that are used in the profession. In groups the individual may play many parts and the group often causes the individual to act differently to the way he or she would in a one-to-one meeting.

Various skills are required both to be a successful group member and to be a group leader or facilitator. Before such skills are discussed, it may be useful to have an overall map of the group process as a means of understanding the stages through which every group, of every sort, seems to pass.

Ward reports/handovers
Case conferences
Ward policy meetings
Unit meetings
Educational groups
Therapy groups
Relaxation groups
Stress management workshops
Study days
Interdisciplinary meetings
Management meetings
Professional issues meetings
Union meetings
Planning meetings
Relatives meetings
Clinical teaching groups

Figure 7.1 Examples of nursing groups

A map of the group process

Figure 7.2 offers such a map, based on the work of Tuckman (1965). He noted that every group passes through four stages in its development and

Stage one: The forming stage
- group members meet
- members hesitantly get to know each other
- trust and disclosure are low
- there is minimal achievement by the group

Stage two: The storming stage
- the group explores relationships between its members
- there is infighting and conflict between group members
- there are tensions between the needs of the individual and the needs of the group

Stage three: The norming stage
- the group establishes rules for itself; both explicit and tacit
- arguments and disagreements are settled
- those who are likely to leave have usually left
- the group becomes cohesive

Stage four: The performing stage
- the group becomes mature and productive
- group members accept individual differences between themselves
- the group can work together
- the group has come of age
  BUT
- there is a danger of stagnation and of 'groupthink'

Figure 7.2   An overview of the group life cycle (after Tuckman, 1965)

life. He described these as the stages of: (a) forming; (b) storming; (c) norming and (d) performing. During stage one, the forming stage, group members meet each other for the first time and attempt to discover what behaviour is and is not required of them. This is a time for testing the water, of discovering other people and for discovering one's role in the group. In many ways, the new member of the group is 'on her best behaviour': the real person has yet to emerge. Henderson and Foster (1991) suggest that at the beginning of a new group, new group members may:

- preserve their sense of safety by silence, intermittent contributions, or a low level of risk taking;
- worry whether they will be included or excluded;
- be cautious about how far to trust the leader and other members with their real reactions;
- feel concern about whether or not they will be liked;
- be more dependent on the group leader for guidance; make choices about the closeness they wish to tolerate by either approach or avoidance of other members and the leader;
- stick with safe topics; address the group leader rather than the other members.

In the storming stage, group members begin to thaw out a little. As a result they characteristically become hostile with one another as they battle to assert themselves and to stamp their personalities on the group. This is the stage of conflict between 'my' needs and wants and those of the group. Often this is a painful period in which there are fights for leadership of the group and attempts at establishing a pecking order. Nurses in the early stages of their nursing education and training, for example, may notice the advent of the storming stage developing once the introductory period in the school or college has been worked through or towards the middle or end of their first year. In this stage, friendships and loyalties are tested and it may be a time when certain individuals either opt out of the group and leave the education and training course or feel pressurized to leave by the group.

Out of the storming stage develops the 'norming' stage, when the group comes to terms with itself and the individuals in it resolve their conflicts to some degree – both personal and interpersonal. In order for the group to function harmoniously, rules, both written and unwritten, are established in the group's resolve to become more cohesive. Members typically get to know one another better and a more trusting, intimate atmosphere develops. Nurse education and training courses when they reach this stage are often perceived as having established themselves by their tutors or lecturers and fellow nurses. The group feels as though it has arrived!

The danger, here, is that such groups will become *too* settled and too complacent. There is also a problem when groups are too readily social-ized into the norms of the institution. In this case, they tend to be readily accepting of what they see and lose a certain critical faculty. It is import-ant that all nurses maintain the ability to think critically and are able to challenge the prevailing practices in the clinical areas in which they work. In most large institutions there develops what has been called an 'organ-izational culture' (Sathe, 1983). That is to say that institutions, as large groups themselves, develop their own norms and seek to initiate new-comers into those norms in order for things to go along much as they have in the past. The new nursing group not only has to develop its own norms but may find itself in conflict or disagreement with the norms of the organizational culture.

The norming stage leads on to the most productive phase of group life: the performing stage. Here, the group has developed a mature collective identity and its members are able to work easily and usefully together. The danger arises, again, in this stage that the group can become com-placent and that new growth is not encouraged. This can be seen in certain clinical environments where everyone has worked together for a considerable period and the group have come to know each other, their habits and behaviours, well. Such a group can become inward looking and reject both new ideas and new members. Consider, for example, some of the reactions that occurred when the nursing process was first intro-duced. A number of people in the profession suggested that: 'we don't need it; we function very well as we are, why change things'. Students arriving in such groups often feel left out or feel that they are intruding. The group that arrives at the performing stage needs to keep itself alert to changes and suggestion from outside of itself. 'Groupthink', the term that is sometimes used to describe the tendency for groups to work as if they were one, closed-minded individual, can occur if the group does not remain in touch and awake to other groups and to new ideas. It could be argued that many nursing groups and perhaps the profession itself has a tendency towards such closed thinking.

This then is a typical cycle through which most groups seem to pass. It may be viewed as a life cycle of the group, and is directly comparable to the life cycle of the individual: it mimics childhood, adolescence, young adulthood and maturity. Thus the life cycle of life as experienced by the individual is played out in the larger arena of the group. Viewed in this light, the group experiences can be valuable for developing further individual awareness. The person who monitors her behaviour and responses in the group can gain insights into themselves through appreciating this correlation between the life cycle of the group and the life cycle of the individual. The nurse in the group may see herself as 'reliving' stages of her own life when she joins that group. The group is perhaps the most potent medium through which to develop self-awareness. In the group both self-disclosure and feedback from others are present – two vital ingredients for awareness.

If the metaphor of the life-cycle of the group is accepted, it will be understood that a group may well reach the point where it has fulfilled its function and the group is disbanded. The cycle has been completed. In nurse education and training this ending of the group life comes naturally at the end of a 3- or 4-year period because the life period for the group has been predetermined by the college, school or examining body. In other groups, however, such a time period may not be so clear-cut and it is important that at periods through any 'performing' period, the group reviews its performance and function. There is little value in continuing the group's existence when the point of its existence has been exhausted. There is nothing worse than belonging to a 'dead' group.

Second to the issue of the group's stages comes the question of the processes that occur during the group's life. All that happens in a group may be divided into two aspects:

(a) content
(b) processes.

Content refers to all that is said and talked about in any given group. Processes are all those things that happen in a group: the dynamics of the group. Such processes occur in all groups of all types. They are more noticeable in small, intimate groups but also frequently occur in professional and work groups. They have been so frequently noted that they are easily described. Figure 7.3 identifies a variety of typical group processes that occur. Recognition of such processes is vital for anyone running groups and it is helpful if group members learn to recognize them. Once again, developing such awareness is part of the larger task of developing personal awareness. It is often useful if the group facilitator holds a discussion about group processes at one of the early meetings of that group. She may also like to invite group members to notice these processes as they occur, thus a sense of group reflexivity occurs. Time can

1. **Pairing**
   Two group members talk to each other rather than to the group.

2. **Projection**
   Group member's blame 'the group', 'the organization' or 'nursing', for the way they are feeling, rather than owning the feeling.

3. **Scapegoating**
   The group picks out one member to act as the person on whom to take out the hostile feelings.

4. **Shutting down**
   A group member cuts his or herself off from the group and becomes isolated a often emotionally distraught.

5. **Rescuing**
   A group member constantly serves as the person who defends other members from attack. Sometimes, the facilitator may *have* to rescue.

6. **Flight**
   The group avoids serious issues by taking avoiding action; talking light-hearte intellectualizing or changing the topic.

Figure 7.3   Examples of group process

then be put aside at regular intervals to discuss the perceived processes. In self-awareness groups, discussion of processes is just as important as the discussion of content. It is regrettable that traditional educational methods have mostly concentrated on the content of courses and study periods at the expense of exploring processes.

Group processes

Typical group processes may thus be described. **Pairing** can be noted when two individuals, usually sitting next to each other, engage in a quiet and often hesitant conversation with each other. The conversation may occur as a series of 'asides', facial expressions and, in the extreme form, in the passing of notes! Pairing is distracting for other group members and may occur as a result of disaffection with the group, insecurity on the part of one or both of the pair involved, boredom or as a means of testing group leadership. Another form of pairing can be seen when two group members form a fairly exclusive relationship and support each other in a determined manner whenever either of them makes a contribution to group affairs and particularly when either of them is under attack from any other group member.

Projection occurs when an individual identifies the group as being responsible for her feelings. The person sees a quality in the group which is, in fact, a quality of her own but of which she is unaware. Thus the individual may say 'this group is hostile and unfriendly' when it is plain to the rest of the group that such a description fits the group member herself. Such projection may arise out of insecurity in the group or out of the individual's own lack of awareness. The process of 'owning' projections and taking responsibility for oneself can be a particularly valuable piece of experiential learning in the group. On the other hand, you have to be careful. Not *everything* that a person says about a group is a projection. Sometimes they are merely describing what is obviously true about the group. So how do you distinguish between a projection and a description? No easy task! Some guidelines that may help here are these:

- a projection is usually only experienced by one person;
- the rest of the group usually disagrees with a projection;
- often the individual comes to recognize her own projections – especially if she is on the lookout for them;
- descriptions are usually corroborated by other group members;
- descriptions do not usually have the 'emotional tone' that can accompany projections.

Scapegoating often occurs during the 'storming' stage of the group. The group looks for someone to blame for the way they are feeling and behaving and chooses a fairly quiet or vulnerable member on whom to vent their feelings. In this sense, scapegoating is a type of collective bullying. Alternatively, the group finds an outside scapegoat and blames 'the organization' or 'the profession' for the circumstances in which it finds itself. This is the 'group beef'. Usually this blaming of outside organizations or bodies is a means of the group avoiding responsibility for itself or a way of avoiding making decisions. Recognition of such scapegoating is part of the group leader's role and identification of it by the group itself can lead to a sense of growing cohesion and personal awareness. Again, though, a word of caution. Sometimes the organization or the profession *is* to blame! It is important to make the distinction.

When a group member becomes **'shut down'** (Heron, 1973), they cut themselves off from the rest of the group, often feeling swamped by it and emotionally fragile. This may be caused by the group member suddenly identifying with a painful experience that is being described by someone else. It may be a response to the general emotional tone of the group or it may be a rejection of the ideas that are being put forward in the group discussion. The skilled group facilitator recognizes such shutting down and helps the individual either to express his feelings or to quietly rejoin the group. There will be occasions, too, when the group member favours a short break from the group. Shutting down often occurs when a group member begins to face important emotional issues that have been previously buried. The shut down person is in crisis. He cannot face his feelings and cannot verbalize how he feels. Working through such a phase must be handled tactfully and sensitively and the person should never be rushed or told that expressing his pent-up feelings would 'do him good'. Sometimes it would: sometimes it wouldn't. The point is that it is the *group member's* place to decide whether or not now is a good time to work through the bottled-up feelings.

The person who **'rescues'** may be a 'compulsive carer'. She may find it easier to defend others from attack than to let those people fend for themselves and learn from the experience. Often rescuing others is a means of avoiding dealing with personal problems: to be seen as the person who always comes to another's aid can serve as a smokescreen for covering unresolved conflicts. It may be that many nurses are compulsive carers. Often it is easier to care for others than it is to care for ourselves. This is fine as far as it goes but constantly caring and rescuing others is a recipe for burnout and emotional exhaustion.

Part of the process of developing self-awareness includes our standing back and enabling others to learn through experience rather than rushing in and helping too quickly. Often the temptation is to protect others from that which we cannot take ourselves. We feel that 'if I can't take it, she can't', forgetting that the other person is a *different* person and blurring the distinction between 'me' and 'you'. As we gain awareness and resilience, we can 'allow' others to live through their own lives without being overprotected or denied the chance to develop their own coping skills. This applies to a wide range of nursing situations: the patient who learns to cope with their anxiety develops the ability to cope with it again; the person who is allowed to live through a certain amount of pain, develops the ability to deal with pain. If we constantly 'rescue' we constantly deny people the ability to develop autonomy.

There are, of course limits to this. The group facilitator has responsibilities towards the members of the group and some judgements have to be made about the degree of rescuing that *the facilitator* can make. As a general rule, she may want to 'rescue' members who are being scapegoated in the early days of the group's development. As the group progresses, she can slowly rescue less and less and allow individuals to fend for themselves more and more.

The group process known as **flight** can be demonstrated in various ways. The group that avoids difficult issues or decisions can be said to be taking flight. The individual group member who is constantly humorous and light-hearted may also be taking flight in humour. The member who always has a theoretical explanation for everything may often be taking flight from feelings. Yet another form of flight is keeping group discussion and meetings on a superficial level, thus deep and more disturbing issues are kept safely at a distance. Identifying and working through flight is a means of helping the group to grow. Self-disclosure occurs more readily when flight is avoided and group members are able to share each other's experiences on an adult-to-adult basis.

Again, this is not to say that all laughter is flight or that the group should always be deep and profound. It is merely to acknowledge that we all escape from facing ourselves: especially in the company of others.

In looking at group processes, it is worth noting that the energy level of any group will fluctuate from time to time just as an individual's energy level will have its peaks and troughs. Part of the development of group life involves living through the periods of low energy and taking advantage of the peaks. Again, the skilful leader and skilful group member will *notice* such fluctuations, take responsibility for them and make adjustments as necessary. When group energy does drop, the following courses of action, by the facilitator, may be appropriate:

(a) sit it out and see what happens
(b) suggest a change of activity
(c) draw the group's attention to the drop in energy
(d) take a short break.

Characteristics of all groups

Finally, small groups have things in common. Dorothy Stock Walker (1987) offers a useful list of the characteristics of groups. The list is as follows:

1. Groups develop particular moods and atmospheres.
2. Shared themes can build up in groups.
3. Groups evolve norms and belief systems.
4. Groups vary in cohesiveness and in the permeability of their boundaries.
5. Groups develop and change their character over a period of time.
6. Persons occupy different positions in groups with respect to power, centrality and being liked and disliked.
7. Individuals in groups sometimes find one or two other persons who are especially important to them because they are similar in some respect to significant persons in the individual's life or to significant aspects of the self.
8. Social comparison can take place in a group.
9. A group is an environment in which persons can observe what others do and say and then observe what happens next.
10. A group is an environment in which persons can receive feedback from others concerning their own behaviour or participation.

Arguably, these characteristics are true of most small groups, from clinical case conferences to learning groups and from therapy groups to discussion groups. Walker's list offers considerable material for discussion with both peers and students and may be a useful starting point for the teaching about groups and group dynamics.

The theoretical and practical issues involved in group work are numerous. The bibliography at the end of this book includes references to other sources that take these and other issues further. It is important that a theoretical and understanding of the nature of groups is essential for anyone who wants to work with groups on a regular and serious basis. Practical experience of groups is vital but this aspect is far easier to manage. As we have noted, we are all involved in group work throughout our professional lives. It is up to us to notice and be aware of the changing patterns and varying natures of those groups. It is through such observations that we learn how other people live and interact together.

In order to highlight some of the aspects of group work, the following exercises explore:

(a) the group experience from the point of view of being a member; and
(b) group facilitation.

These exercises may be followed through systematically or specific ones may be chosen to highlight or experience a particular aspect of group work. It is often useful if these exercises are preceded by one or two 'icebreaker' exercises in order to help the group to relax and settle into the atmosphere of the session.

Exercises in group membership

In the following exercises, a clear aim is offered for each. This group may be told of this objective before carrying out the exercise or, the group may carry out the exercise and make what they will of it. As we noted earlier, behavioural objectives are not particularly helpful in the experiential learning field: the whole focus of the enterprise is on the individual's subjective experience. Herein lies a conundrum. On the one hand, the facilitator clearly has something in mind when he suggests an activity. On the other, he is keen that group members learn what *they* need to learn from it. Sometimes to disclose an aim is to pre-empt the group's own learning from experience. Instead, when the aim is disclosed, the group helps to ensure that a self-fulfilling prophesy occurs: the group works towards achieving that aim. There is no easy answer to this. Probably a compromise is best. When it seems necessary to offer a rationale for a particular activity, disclose the aim. When the need is not so great, suggest the activity but not the aim.

Exercises similar to and variants of the following exercises may be found in a variety of sources: see, for example, Stevens, 1971; Heron, 1973; Canfield and Wells, 1976; Kagan *et al.*, 1986; Arnold and Boggs, 1989; Burnard, 1989b; Heron, 1989a.

As was the case with the exercises in the previous chapter, it is important that participation in the group exercises is voluntary. If any member asks not to take part, such a request should be honoured without question. The member who chooses not to take part in this way may usefully serve as a process observer and offer feedback to the group once the exercise has been completed. It is notable that some people find group activities difficult and whilst they are quite happy to take part in pairs activities such as those described in the last chapter, they are less happy talking in front of the whole group.

Exercise 30

Aim of the exercise: To explore the relationships and perceptions of group members.
Group size: Any number from 6 to 20.
Time required: About 40 minutes.
Materials and/or environment required: A large, comfortable room and a circle of straight-backed chairs.

Process

1. The facilitator explains the exercise as follows. Each group member arranges the rest of the group in order to form a family (e.g. 'David is my father, Sue my sister, Sian my cousin . . .' and so on).
2. When each group member has developed a family in this way, the facilitator develops a discussion about the activity.

Evaluation

The facilitator may want to ask:

- What did you feel about being part of someone else's 'family'?
- What did you think about the positions you were given?
- What does all this say about our relationships with each other?

Notes

A variation on this activity is for one 'family' to stay intact and to 'stay in role'. Relationships between 'family' members is then explored.

Exercise 31

Aim of the exercise: To develop group relationships and to highlight the occurrence of group processes.
Group size: Any number from 6 to 20.
Time required: Between 1 and 2 hours.
Materials and/or environment required: A large, comfortable room and a circle of straight-backed chairs.

Process

1. The group facilitator invites the group to discuss one of the following topics:
   (a) the caring relationship in nursing
   (b) the qualities of friendship
   (c) our relationships with each other.
2. The group is asked to observe the following ground rules (which may be displayed on a large sheet of paper or given to the group in the form of a handout):
   - Speak in the 'first person' (use 'I' rather than 'you', 'we' or 'people'. Thus, 'I am angry at the moment' rather than 'You always get angry when people treat you like that, don't you?').
   - Speak directly to other people, rather than *about* them. (Thus: 'I don't agree with you' in preference to 'I don't agree with what Gary says').
   - Make statements rather than asking questions (e.g. 'I'm enjoying this', rather than 'Is everyone enjoying doing this?').
   - Avoid theorizing and explaining other people's behaviour (e.g. Avoid making statements such as: 'I think what James is really trying to say is . . .' or 'What Ali really thinks is . . .').

3. The facilitator indicates to the group *every* time a rule is broken and invites the person to rephrase their statement.
4. After 1 hour has elapsed, the rules are dropped and the facilitator convenes a discussion on the effects of using the rules.

Evaluation

The facilitator may want to ask:

- What was the experience like?
- Why did no one break the rules?
- What was it like when you did?

Notes

This set of rules is a useful one for enhancing clear communication and may be used as a set of 'ground rules' for a workshop or study day. Also, the group may be encouraged to monitor the ground rules themselves. It is always interesting when someone intentionally flouts all of them!

Exercise 32

Aim of the exercise: To encourage attention to the group and listening between members of the group.
Group size: Any number from 6 to 20.
Time required: Between 1 and 2 hours.
Materials and/or environment required: A large, comfortable room and a circle of straight-backed chairs.

Process

1. The group facilitator invites the group to discuss one of the following topics:
    (a) the problems of becoming self-aware
    (b) how I stop myself from becoming self-aware
    (c) any other topic.
2. The facilitator explains that after one member has spoken, any other member who wishes to speak must first *summarise* what the previous speaker has said. They may then make their own contribution.
3. This activity is carried on for about 1 hour and the group then reconvenes. The facilitator invokes a discussion on the exercise, without the summarizing rule.

Evaluation

The facilitator may want to ask:

- What problems did you have with this exercise?
- How well do you *normally* listen to other people in groups?

Notes

This exercise can also be used as a listening exercise in pairs. In this case, one person in the pair must always summarize what the other had said before making their own contribution. A similar approach was originally used by Carl Rogers as a method for developing client-centred counselling skills (Kirschenbaum, 1979).

Exercise 33

Aim of the exercise: To explore group processes without non-verbal cues.
Group size: Any number from 6 to 20.
Time required: About 40 minutes.
Materials and/or environment required: A large, comfortable room and a circle of straight-backed chairs.

Process

1. The facilitator invites the group to turn their chairs around so that they all sit facing outwards, in a closed circle.
2. The facilitator then initiates a discussion on the topic of 'the importance of verbal and non-verbal communication'.
3. After 20 minutes, the group is asked to turn their chairs back round and to share their experiences.

Evaluation

The facilitator may want to ask:

- What did it feel like *not being able to see* the other members of the group? What are the advantages of not being able to see non-verbal behaviour?

Notes

This activity can be carried out in pairs to explore effective ways of communicating on the telephone. In this version, each pair sits back to back and holds a 'telephone conversation'. It may be used to explore breaking bad news over the telephone.

Exercise 34

Aim of the exercise: To experiment with the concept of shared leadership.
Group size: Any number from 6 to 20.
Time required: About 2 hours.
Materials and/or environment required: A large, comfortable room and a circle of straight-backed chairs. A small cushion.

Process

1. The group facilitator describes the process of this activity as follows:
    (a) Only the person holding the cushion may talk.
    (b) A person wishing to say something must indicate that they want the cushion but must not speak until they hold it.
2. The facilitator places the cushion in the centre of the circle and invites the group to discuss one of the following topics, whilst observing the rules of the exercise:
    (a) nursing models
    (b) nursing theory
    (c) nursing research
    (d) the idea of a leaderless group
    (e) any other topic.
3. After 1 hour, the facilitator suggests dropping the rules and invokes a discussion on the exercise.

Evaluation

The facilitator may want to ask:

- Would it be possible to have a leaderless group in any other circumstances? Why did no one hold on to the cushion?

Notes

An interesting variation on this activity is for the facilitator not to suggest a topic for the exercise but to allow the group discussion to evolve spontaneously. This version is only recommended where group members know each other fairly well.

Exercise 35

Aim of the exercise: To explore the effects of silence in the group.
Group size: Any number from 6 to 20.
Time required: About 40 minutes.
Materials and/or environment required: A large, comfortable room and a circle of straight-backed chairs.

Process

1. The group facilitator invites the group to remain completely silent for 10 minutes.
2. The facilitator breaks the silence at the end of the 10-minute period and invokes a discussion on the feelings and experiences of the group during the silent period.

Evaluation

The facilitator may want to ask:

- How can silence in a group be dealt with?
- How do *you* normally cope with silences?

Notes

This activity is best carried out with a group of people that know each other fairly well.

Exercise 36

Aim of the exercise: To explore group feelings in a symbolic format.
Group size: Any number from 6 to 20.
Time required: Between 1 and $1\frac{1}{2}$ hours.
Materials and/or environment required: A large, comfortable room and a circle of straight-backed chairs. Large sheets of white paper. Paints, pastels, or coloured pencils for each person.

Process

1. The group facilitator asks each group member to draw an abstract or figurative picture of the group in any style that the person chooses. The facilitator emphasizes that no particular artistic experience is required.
2. On completion of the pictures, each member presents her picture to the group.
3. The facilitator then invites discussion on the significance of the pictures and invites comments on any similarities and differences between the various pictures.

Evaluation

The facilitator may want to ask:

- What do these symbols *mean*? (It is important that people are allowed to interpret *their own* pictures and that the facilitator does not rush to do this for them.)

Notes

The pictures may be displayed on the wall as a backdrop to a workshop or study day. It is also interesting to repeat this exercise with the same group at a later date and to compare the pictures from each occasion.

Exercise 37

Aim of the exercise: To explore self-disclosure and risk-taking.
Group size: Any number from 6 to 20.
Time required: Between 40 minutes and 1 hour.

Materials and/or environment required: A large, comfortable room and a circle of straight-backed chairs.

Process

1. The group facilitator invites each group member in turn to complete some of the following sentences. A 'round' of the group is completed before moving on to the next item.
   (a) I am feeling ...
   (b) What I am not saying at the moment is ...
   (c) I could shock the group if I ...
   (d) What I like most about this group is ...
   (e) What I like least about this group is ...
   (f) The topic that I find most difficult to discuss is ...
   (g) I would be happier if this group ...
   (h) If I could be anywhere else at the moment I would choose to be ...
   (g) If I had to change places with a famous person, I would change places with ...
2. After the rounds have been completed the facilitator invites a free discussion on the exercise.

Evaluation

The facilitator may want to ask:

- What was it like waiting for your turn?
- Were any of the questions or statements more difficult than others?

Notes

The facilitator may invite the group to make up their own sentences for completion and also to facilitate the group whilst those sentences are being completed.

Exercise 38

Aim of the exercise: To explore similarities and differences between group members.
Group size: Any number from 6 to 20.
Time required: Between 40 minutes and 1 hour.
Materials and/or environment required: A large, comfortable room and a circle of straight-backed chairs.

Process

1. The facilitator invites group members, in turn, to say:
   (a) who they feel is *most* like them in the group
   (b) who is most *different* to them in the group.

2. The facilitator asks that group members do not give a reason for their choice at this stage.
3. When each member has had her turn, the facilitator invites a discussion on the perceptions of group members.

Evaluation

The facilitator may want to ask:

- What was it like being compared in this way?
- Where there any surprises?

Notes

It is important that the facilitator makes it clear that what is being asked is who is *most different* to the person concerned and not who the other person *least likes*. This is a considerable shift in emphasis.

Exercise 39

Aim of the exercise: To explore group norms.
Group size: Any number from 6 to 20.
Time required: About 1 hour.
Materials and/or environment required: A large, comfortable room and a circle of straight-backed chairs. Large sheets of paper and pens.

Process

1. The facilitator hands out sheets of paper to each member of the group and asks them to draw three columns on the sheet.
2. Each person is invited to jot down ideas in the three columns as follows:
   (a) the norms that operate in this group
   (b) the norms that operate in my home
   (c) the norms that operate in this school or college of nursing.
3. After 20 minutes, the facilitator reconvenes the group and invites feedback on the activity. The sheets are displayed in the centre of the group.

Evaluation

The facilitator may want to ask:

- Are there great differences between norms in the three settings?
- If so, why is this the case?
- How did these norms come into being?
- Why?

Notes

Other norms can be explored in this way: e.g.

(a) personal norms
(b) church norms
(c) ward norms
(d) secondary school norms
(e) norms in different classes in the school or college
(f) societal norms.

Exercise 40

Aim of the exercise: To share positive, formative experiences in a group setting.
Group size: Any number from 6 to 20.
Time required: Between 1 and $1\frac{1}{2}$ hours.
Materials and/or environment required: A large, comfortable room and a circle of straight-backed chairs.

Process

1. The facilitator invites the group to sit in silence for 2 minutes and to recall three positive, formative experiences from their childhood or up to the present time.
2. Group members then share those experiences with the group.
3. The group facilitator invites a discussion on formative experiences.

Evaluation

The facilitator may want to ask:

- *How* were these formative?
- Did you find that you thought of others but did not disclose them? (This should not be an invitation for further disclosure but can help people to become aware of what goes on 'just below the surface'.)

Notes

A challenging exercise for groups that know each other really well is for each member to also recall three *negative* experiences. If this format is used, it is recommended that the plan is as follows:

(a) the group members disclose and discuss *negative* experiences and then
(b) the group members disclose and discuss *positive* ones.

In this format the group closes on a positive note.

Exercise 41

Aim of the exercise: To explore members' perceptions of their position in the group.

Group size: Any number from 6 to 20.
Time required: About 1 hour.
Materials and/or environment required: A large, comfortable room and a circle of straight-backed chairs.

Process

1. The group facilitator invites each member in turn to report to the group how they imagine the rest of the group sees them (e.g. 'I imagine that the group sees me as a fairly optimistic person with a lot to say and who sometimes talks too much').
2. After all members have had their turn, the group facilitator invites feedback to individual members, from the group.

Evaluation

The facilitator may want to ask:

• What were the difficulties with this activity?
• Did you enjoy it?

Exercise 42

Aim of the exercise: To explore self-disclosure and group decision making.
Group size: Any number from 6 to 20.
Time required: Between 40 minutes and 1 hour.
Materials and/or environment required: A large, comfortable room and a circle of straight-backed chairs. Sheets of lined paper for each person.

Process

1. The facilitator invites each group member to write down three topics that they would find very difficult to discuss. No further instructions are given.
2. When all group members have finished writing, the facilitator invites the group to decide democratically what is to be done with the sheets of paper. They may, for instance. decide to:
   (a) tear up the sheets
   (b) read out the items on the sheets
   (c) allow individuals to modify their sheets
   (d) pile up the sheets in the middle of the group and pick up someone else's sheet and then read that sheet aloud
   (e) recall the sheets and rewrite them
   (f) disclose one item from the list.
3. After the process has been completed, the facilitator invokes a discussion on the exercise.

Evaluation

The facilitator may want to ask:

- Did *your* ideas about what should happen to the sheets coincide with what was decided?
- If not, how do you feel about that?
- What could you have done to change the decision?

Notes

A variation on this exercise is to invite people to jot down three things about themselves that they would find difficult to talk about. An important point about this activity is that *any* individual who wishes to withdraw what they have written should reserve the right to do so at any time. This rule should override the decision made in the exercise.

Exercise 43

Aim of the exercise: To experience being asked questions by other group members and self-disclosing to the group.
Group size: Any number from 6 to 20.
Time required: Between 1 and 2 hours.
Materials and/or environment required: A large, comfortable room and a circle of straight-backed chairs.

Process

1. The facilitator explains that each group member, including the facilitator, will spend 3 minutes being asked questions on any topic by the rest of the group. The individual in the 'hot seat' may choose to 'pass' on any question that he or she does not wish to answer.
2. One member volunteers to go first.
3. At the end of the 3 minutes, that person nominates another member of the group to take the hot seat until everyone in the group has had a turn.
4. At any time, a group member may choose to 'pass' on the whole activity and not take their place in the hot seat.
5. The facilitator should consider not passing on any question when it is their turn to take the hot seat.
6. At the end of the process, the facilitator invites a discussion on the group's experience of the exercise.

Evaluation

The facilitator may want to ask:

- What sort of questions were asked mostly: open or closed?
- What motivated you to ask the questions that you did?
- What does all this tell you about the process of asking questions.

What the facilitator should NOT ask is why individuals 'passed' on certain questions.

Notes

This activity has numerous applications. It can, for instance, be used with questions focused around a particular topic, as a revision aid. For example:

(a) nursing theory
(b) aspects of anatomy and physiology
(c) legal aspects of nursing
(d) ethical issues in nursing.

It can also be used in a shortened version as an icebreaker. Here, the time for questions is limited to $1\frac{1}{2}$ minutes for each person.

Exercise 44

Aim of the exercise: To explore the use of touch in a group setting.
Group size: Any number from 6 to 20.
Time required: Between 40 minutes and 1 hour.
Materials and/or environment required: A large, comfortable room and a circle of straight-backed chairs.

Process

1. The facilitator invites the group to put on blindfolds or to close their eyes and keep them closed.
2. The facilitator then instructs the group to wander silently around the room.
3. As group members meet, they are invited to identify each other by touch alone. Once correct identification has been made, the person who has been identified can acknowledge who he or she is.
4. After all group members have be so identified, the facilitator encourages the group to re-form and a discussion is held on the experience of the exercise.

Evaluation

The facilitator may want to ask:

• What was it like to wander round blindfolded?
• Did you *hope* to identify certain people?
• Were there any surprises?

Notes

The facilitator should remain unblindfolded in order to ensure that group members do not hurt themselves through collisions with people or objects.

A variation on this activity is the traditional 'blind walk'. Here, group members pair off and one of each pair is blindfolded and then led around by their partner to experience what it is like to be deprived of one sense. The pairs are encouraged to wander around outside the building, to attempt, carefully, the negotiation of stairs, to encourage the blindfolded person to touch objects, buildings, surfaces and so forth. A variant of *this* activity is for the blindfolded person only to be 'minded' by the other person. In other words, the pair wander round in silence and the blindfolded person does not hold the arm of the other person. The blindfolded person is apparently on their own. Both of these activities are powerful ones that are worthy of considerable discussion afterwards.

Exercise 45

Aim of the exercise: To identify relative roles and relationship of members of the group.
Group size: Any number from 6 to 20.
Time required: Between 30 minutes and 1 hour.
Materials and/or environment required: A large, comfortable room and a circle of straight-backed chairs.

Process

1. The facilitator invites the group to stand up and stand along an imaginary line, in the position that they feel they occupy in the group.
2. The facilitator may offer suggestions about the end points of the line: e.g.
   (a) quiet ... talkative
   (b) extrovert ... introvert
   (c) submissive ... dominant.
   Alternatively, the facilitator may leave the group to decide on its own criteria.
3. When the line has been completed, the facilitator invites individual members to make changes to the order of the group as they see fit.
4. When the process has been completed, the facilitator invites the group to sit down and to discuss the implications of the line-up.

Evaluation

The facilitator may want to ask:

- Did you 'allow' yourself to be placed in line or did you *decide*?
- Are there any other criteria for sorting people in this group?

Exercise 46

Aim of the exercise: To explore individual group members' perceptions of themselves.

Group size: Any number from 6 to 20.
Time required: Between 40 minutes and 1 hour.
Materials and/or environment required: A large, comfortable room and a circle of straight-backed chairs.

Process

1. The facilitator invites group members to think of a household object OR a piece of music OR a book.
2. Group members are then invited to describe themselves in turn as though they *were that object*, in the first person (e.g. 'armchair': ' I am soft and large and often get sat on by other people ...').
3. When each member of the group has had a turn the facilitator leads a discussion on the exercise.

Evaluation

The facilitator may want to ask:

- Can you describe yourselves as objects that *other* people chose?
- What did you make of the descriptions?

Notes

As a variation on this activity, the facilitator may choose a category of item for each group member, thus:

(a) Imagine you are a piece of music ... what piece of music are you? Describe yourself as that.
(b) Imagine you are a piece of furniture ... what piece of furniture are you? Describe yourself as that.
(c) Imagine you are an animal ... what animal? Describe yourself as that.

Other categories that may be suggested are: a country, a book, a town, a river, a statue, a period in history, another person, a car, a building and so on.

Exercise 47

Aim of the exercise: To explore spatial relationships between group members.
Group size: Any number from 6 to 20.
Time required: About 40 minutes.
Materials and/or environment required: A large, comfortable room and a circle of straight-backed chairs.

Process

1. The facilitator invites the group to wander round the room and to take time in finding the exact spot where they want to sit. Allow them to take plenty of time to do this.

2. From these positions, the group members are invited to share their thoughts on the significance of their positions.

Evaluation

The facilitator may want to ask:

- How did you choose *that* spot?

Notes

This activity may also be carried out with group members wearing blindfolds which are only taken off once everyone is seated. A discussion can then be held on the relative positions of everyone in the room.

Exercise 48

Aim of the exercise: To share positive feelings for individual members and to enhance group cohesiveness.
Group size: Any number from 6 to 20.
Time required: Between 1 and $1\frac{1}{2}$ hours.
Materials and/or environment required: A large, comfortable room and a circle of straight-backed chairs.

Process

1. The facilitator invites each group member to listen to a 'round' of validating comments from each other group member. If required, the incomplete sentence 'The things I like most about you are . . .' may be used.
2. The group member being validated in this way receives the round without comment.
3. When all the group members have taken part, the facilitator invokes a discussion on the exercise.

Evaluation

The facilitator may want to ask:

- Did you all *agree* with the comments that were made about you?
- What was it like to receive feedback of this sort?
- How skilled are you in telling people that you like them?

Notes

If group members know each other very well, a challenging exercise can be to invite *negative* feedback in the same format as above. The facilitator should ask that such feedback be given tactfully and supportively. This version should be used with care and only with the complete agreement of each member of the group. As with all the activities, individual members may reserve the right to opt out at any time during the activity.

Exercise 49

Aim of the exercise: To experience self and peer assessment in a group.
Group size: Any number from 6 to 20.
Time required: Between 1 and 2 hours.
Materials and/or environment required: A large, comfortable room and a circle of straight-backed chairs.

Process

1. The facilitator invites each group member to assess her personal weaknesses and strengths and to disclose these to the group.
2. Following this disclosure, the group member invites feedback of perceived weaknesses and strengths from other group members. Thus, in this stage, the rest of the group tell the individual about their perceptions of that individual.
3. When each member has both offered assessment and received feedback, the facilitator invites a free discussion on the process.

Evaluation

The facilitator may want to ask:

• What were the differences between your assessment of yourself and that of the group?

Notes

The process can also be used at the end of a learning session as a means of self- and peer evaluation. It is important that assessment and feedback are always offered in the order:

(a) weaknesses and
(b) strengths

so that the process ends on a positive note.

Exercise 50

Aim of the exercise: To close a group.
Group size: Any number from 6 to 20.
Time required: 10 minutes.

Materials and/or environment required: A large, comfortable room and a circle of straight-backed chairs.

Process

1. The facilitator invites the group to stand up, to move into a close, standing circle and to put their arms around the shoulders of the people standing next to them.
2. Group members are then encouraged to share thoughts about the day's activities or about each other.
3. After a few minutes, the group disbands without further discussion.

Exercises in group facilitation

The term 'facilitator' has been used throughout this section of the book to describe the person who initiates group activity or who leads the group in some way. The lecturer or tutor running such a group, whose aim is developing self-awareness, is a facilitator, as is the student nurse who sets up a learning group for patients in a clinical setting. The nurse who acts as facilitator needs to make some consideration about how to fulfil that role prior to setting up the group in question. Henderson and Foster (1991) offer a useful list of what they call *group leadership functions*. They suggest that the facilitator or leader of a group should involve him or herself in:

- being clear about objectives;
- selecting an appropriate group size for the group purpose;
- teaching group-process skills to members if necessary (taking turns, listening to others, building on their ideas);
- proposing and promoting ways of behaving that increase trust, acceptance, mutual support, challenge and empower;
- promoting participating by inviting members to contribute;
- interrupting monopolizers without attacking them;
- observing and monitoring group behaviour;
- facilitating emotional expressing, where appropriate;
- encouraging members to experiment with new behaviour or ideas;
- modelling how to give positive and negative feedback.

This leads on to the notion of *facilitator style*: the 'way of being' with a group that the facilitator chooses from a range of possibilities.

Facilitator style

John Heron (1989b) has described six dimensions of what he calls 'facilitator style' that may help here. Those dimensions are outlined in Figure 7.4. It is not suggested that a potential facilitator must use one particular aspect of a dimension rather than another but rather that

Directive		**Non-directive**
The facilitator clearly directs the group	*or*	The facilitator encourages the group to make decisions for itself
Interpretative		**Non-interpretative**
The facilitator offers the group interpretations of its behaviour	*or*	The facilitator encourages the group to interpret its own behaviour
Confronting		**Non-confronting**
The facilitator challenges the group	*or*	The facilitator encourages the group to challenge itself
Cathartic		**Non-cathartic**
The facilitator encourages the release of emotions in the group	*or*	The facilitator steers the group into less emotional territory
Structuring		**Un-structuring**
The facilitator uses activities, exercises and games to bring structure to the group	*or*	The facilitator works with the group in a less formal way
Disclosing		**Non-disclosing**
The facilitator shares his/her own thoughts, feelings and experiences with the group	*or*	The facilitator keeps his/her own thoughts, feelings and experiences to herself

Figure 7.4   Dimensions of facilitator style (after Heron, 1989b)

such a decision will arise out of the *type* of group that is to be facilitated. The analysis of facilitator styles is particularly useful in identifying the *range* of possible options open to the group leader.

The sorts of questions that may be asked in relation to the six dimension before attempting to facilitate a group are as follows:

1. Does this group need to be *led* or can it be free flowing and open ended? (the directive–non-directive dimension).
2. Do I need to explain what is happening in the group? Do I need to offer theories and frameworks for understanding what is going on or can the group 'explain itself'? (the interpretative–non-interpretative dimension).
3. Do I need to challenge the group and to point out rigidities and repetitions in the group and individual behaviour or can I let the group sort these issues out for themselves? (the confronting–non-confronting dimension).
4. Will I be able to handle the expression of laughter, tears, anger or fear or will I need to divert it through lighter topics? (the cathartic–non cathartic dimension).
5. Should I use exercises, games, plans and set procedures to bring structure to the group or should I let the group organize itself? (the structuring–unstructuring dimension.)
6. Am I going to let the group share my own thoughts and feelings as they occur or will I play a more neutral role? (the disclosing–non disclosing dimension).

Sometimes the *aim and purpose* of the group meeting will help to determine the style to be used. Consider, for example, the following types of groups. What would be examples of *inappropriate* styles of group facilitation in each one?

- A planning meeting
- A group therapy meeting
- A meeting of friends in the pub
- A political meeting
- A discussion group in the school or college

The nurse, lecturer, tutor or trainer who considers these issues is developing the conscious use of self alluded to earlier. If these issues are clarified the facilitator will be in a better position to act knowingly rather that blindly or unawarely. We cannot *change* our behaviour until we *know* what our behaviour is. To go to a group prepared in this way is to have considered the needs of the group. Not all groups are the same and not all groups will require the same sorts of facilitation.

Generally, a useful rule for working with self-awareness groups is to begin with a directive, structured and lightly confronting approach and gradually to help the group take more and more responsibility for itself. As the group progresses, the facilitator is, one the one hand, increasingly non-directive, unstructuring and non-confronting and on the other, increasingly cathartic and disclosing. Whether or not to be interpretative of other people's behaviour is a moot point. As a rule (and adopting a phenomenological point of view) such interpretations are probably best left to the individual to make. It is often better to be *descriptive* rather than interpretative. Consider this difference in the following example.

A group is discussing a point which causes one member to begin to move around in her seat and to stop talking. The group facilitator who is being *descriptive says*: ' I notice that you are quieter than you were and that you are shifting around in your seat quite a lot.' The group facilitator who is *interpretative* says: ' I think you are finding this discussion a bit difficult and that it is making you anxious.' The description allows the group member to interpret her own behaviour and to report her own feelings as she chooses. The interpretation pre-empts the individual's perception of what she is doing and why she is doing it.

Figure 7.5 summarizes these points about the changing emphasis of group facilitation.

The general points that may be made about the nurse, tutor, lecturer or trainer who is facilitating a well-established group is that he should not over-direct the group but should allow it to develop for itself. He should not depend too much on structured exercises but allow the group to develop its own structure. He should consider allowing the free expression of emotion where it is appropriate and be prepared not to rush in and try to rescue or 'explain' people's emotions to them. He should not rush to interpret other people's behaviour but encourage individuals to make their own sense of what happens to them. These points are generally in line with the philosophy of experiential learning so far discussed (although the list contains rather too may 'shoulds' and 'nots' for my liking!). Experiential learning is, after all, about the reflection on personal

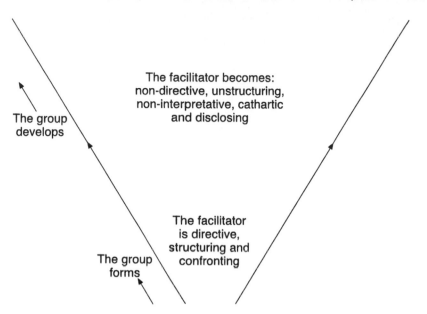

Figure 7.5   Appropriate styles of group facilitation for self-awareness groups

experience and about the personal ownership and transformation of meaning. We can never create meaning for other people: in the end each person finds it for himself.

The exercises that follow allow for a systematic investigation of the six dimensions of facilitator style. They may be used progressively and in order so that a range of facilitation skills is built up. Alternatively, one or two may be selected to develop a particular aspect of facilitation. As with Heron's (1989a) Six Category Intervention Analysis (out of which the dimensions were developed), the skilled facilitator is one who can freely choose and intelligently use any aspect of the six dimensions.

It is possible to combine the use of the styles of facilitation with the skills learned through the use of Six Category Intervention Analysis. Figure 7.6 illustrates the relationship between these two models. The styles of facilitation model outlines the general considerations that a group facilitator must make: the category analysis equips them with a range of specific *group interventions*.

In the end, both the styles model and the category analysis have wide applications in teaching and learning, nursing practice, organizing and running meetings, clinical supervision, research supervision and the development of interpersonal or human skills.

Exercise 51

Aim of the exercise: To exercise a directive style of group facilitation.
Group size: Any number from 6 to 20.

Stage one: Setting up a group

Question: What *general* consideration do I need to make about the group
facilitation before I start running a group?
Answer: Consult dimensions of facilitator style and choose from the
following dimensions:

Directive style ──────── Non-directive style
Interpretative style ──────── Non-interpretative style
Confronting style ──────── Non-confronting style
Cathartic style ──────── Non-cathartic style
Structuring style ──────── Unstructuring style
Disclosing style ──────── Non-disclosing style

Consider, also:

1. Stages of group formation: 2. Group dynamics:
  —forming   —pairing
  —storming   —rescuing
  —norming   —scapegoating etc.
  —performing

3. Environmental considerations:
  —seating
  —lighting
  —ventilation etc.

Stage two: Facilitating the group

Question: What *specific* interventions can I make when I facilitate the group?
Answer: Consult Six Category Intervention Analysis and choose from the
following interventions:

• Prescriptive interventions
• Informative interventions
• Confronting interventions
• Cathartic interventions
• Catalytic interventions
• Supportive interventions

Figure 7.6   The relationship between the dimensions of facilitator style and Six
Category Intervention Analysis

Time required: About 1 hour.
Materials and/or environment required: A large, comfortable room and a
circle of straight-backed chairs.

Process

1. The facilitator decides upon a subject for discussion by the group and keeps the
group to the topic.
2. After half an hour the facilitator sums up and closes the discussion.
3. The facilitator self-evaluates her own performance by describing the short-
comings and strengths of her facilitation to the group.
4. The facilitator invites peer evaluation by asking for feedback from the group on
her performance. It is helpful if group members first say what they *did not like*
about her facilitation and then what they *liked* about it.

Notes

In this and all the activities designed to exercise particular facilitation skills, the term 'facilitator' can either mean the tutor, lecturer or other nursing professional or it can refer to the student in a group who is learning to facilitate groups.

Exercise 52

Aim of the exercise: To exercise a non-directive style of group facilitation.
Group size: Any number from 6 to 20.
Time required: About 1 hour.
Materials and/or environment required: A large, comfortable room and a circle of straight-backed chairs.

Process

1. The facilitator asks the group what they would like to talk about and allows a free-ranging discussion to develop, making no attempt to keep the group to the topic but allowing the discussion to evolve as the group wishes. The facilitator should try to restrict his interventions to the following:
   (a) open questions;
   (b) reflections;
   (c) empathy building statements.
2. After half an hour the facilitator closes the discussion without summary.
3. The facilitator self-evaluates his own performance by describing the shortcomings and strengths of his facilitation to the group.
4. The facilitator invites peer evaluation by asking for feedback from the group on his performance. It is helpful if group members first say what they *did not like* about his facilitation and then what they *liked* about it.

Exercise 53

Aim of the exercise: To exercise an interpretative style of group facilitation.
Group size: Any number from 6 to 20.
Time required: About 1 hour.
Materials and/or environment required: A large, comfortable room and a circle of straight-backed chairs.

Process

1. The facilitator either decides on a topic for discussion or negotiates a topic with the group.
2. During the discussion, the facilitator offers possible explanations for the behaviour, ideas or feelings of group members.

3. After half an hour, the facilitator sums up both the content of the group discussion and attempts to shed light on the process that occurred.
4. The facilitator self-evaluates her own performance by describing the short-comings and strengths of her facilitation to the group.
5. The facilitator invites peer evaluation by asking for feedback from the group on her performance. It is helpful if group members first say what they *did not like* about her facilitation and then what they *liked* about it.

Notes

The facilitator may want to choose from a variety of theoretical frame-works from which to interpret the group's behaviour, thoughts, feelings or ideas. A short list of such theoretical frameworks might include:

(a) psychodynamic theory;
(b) behavioural theory;
(c) humanistic theory;
(d) sociological theory;
(e) theological theory;
(f) transactional analytic theory;
(g) gestalt theory etc.

The problem with this approach is whether the facilitator ever knows enough about a theoretical framework to make an informed interpreta-tion. Thus the accent in the text above on inviting the group members to make sense of *their own* experience wherever possible. A central tenet of this book is that we are the experts on our own behaviour, thoughts and feelings.

Exercise 54

Aim of the exercise: To exercise a non-interpretative style of group facil-itation.
Group size: Any number from 6 to 20.
Time required: About 1 hour.
Materials and/or environment required: A large, comfortable room and a circle of straight-backed chairs.

Process

1. The facilitator either decides upon a topic for discussion or negotiates the topic with the group.
2. During the discussion, the facilitator invites possible explanations for the be-haviour, thoughts, feelings or ideas from the group members. The facilitator pays particular attention to group members' interpretations of *their own* behav-iour, thoughts and feelings. He offers no interpretations of *his own* but can report to the group on his own thoughts and feelings.
3. After half an hour, the facilitator draws the discussion to a close and invites the group to sum up the main issues that have been discussed.

4. The facilitator self-evaluates his own performance by describing the short-comings and strengths of his facilitation to the group.
5. The facilitator invites peer evaluation by asking for feedback from the group on his performance. It is helpful if group members first say what they *did not like* about his facilitation and then what they *liked* about it.

Exercise 55

Aim of the Exercise: To exercise a confronting style of group facilitation.
Group size: Any number from 6 to 20.
Time required: About 1 hour.
Materials and/or environment required: A large, comfortable room and a circle of straight-backed chairs.

Process

1. The facilitator either decides upon a topic for discussion or negotiates a topic with the group.
2. During the discussion, the facilitator draws attention to any of the following:
   (a) errors of logic in a group member's argument
   (b) mismatches between what a group member is *saying* and her facial expression or 'body language'
   (c) repetitions
   (d) errors of fact
   (e) any tendency for a group member to generalize from a single case
   (f) a silent member of the group.
3. After half and hour the facilitator draws the discussion to a close and sums up the content and process of the discussion.
4. The facilitator self-evaluates her own performance by describing the short-comings and strengths of her facilitation to the group.
5. The facilitator invites peer evaluation by asking for feedback from the group on her performance. It is helpful if group members first say what they *did not like* about her facilitation and then what they *liked* about it.

Exercise 56

Aim of the exercise: To exercise a non-confronting style of group leadership.
Group size: Any number from 6 to 20.
Time required: About 1 hour.
Materials and/or environment required: A large, comfortable room and a circle of straight-backed chairs.

Process

1. The facilitator either decides upon a topic for discussion or negotiates a topic with the group.

2. Before commencing the discussion, the facilitator invites the group to be awake to the occurrence of any errors of logic, repetitive behaviour, contradictions and so forth.
3. During the discussion, the facilitator makes no attempt to confront the group or individual members but allows the group to make its own confrontations.
4. The facilitator self-evaluates his own performance by describing the short-comings and strengths of his facilitation to the group.
5. The facilitator invites peer evaluation by asking for feedback from the group on his performance. It is helpful if group members first say what they *did not like* about his facilitation and then what they *liked* about it.

Notes

It is often a good idea to run these activities one after the other as a series of pairs. Thus, the confronting activity is followed by the non-confronting activity, both led by the same person. Following a pair of exercises, both the facilitator and the group can decide which style they prefer and suggest when one style would be more appropriately used than the other.

Exercise 57

Aim of the exercise: To exercise a cathartic style of group facilitation.
Group size: Any number from 6 to 20.
Time required: About 2 hours.
Materials and/or environment required: A large, comfortable room and a circle of straight-backed chairs.

Process

1. The facilitator invites the group to embark on a discussion about personal or emotional issues. Clearly such a topic must be negotiated with the group.
2. The facilitator makes it clear at the outset that group members are free to express any feelings as they occur.
3. During the discussion, the facilitator tries to restrict her interventions to the following:
    (a) she invites particular group members to literally describe a place that they have been talking about that seems to evoke emotion;
    (b) she asks particular group members to note how they are feeling and to *exaggerate* the way that they are feeling;
    (c) she encourages particular group members to exaggerate hand movements and gestures that they make and then asks 'What's the feeling that goes with that ...?'.
4. After about three-quarters of an hour, the facilitator draws the discussion to a close and to a lighter level as necessary. Such lightening of the atmosphere may be achieved by one of the following mini exercises:
    (a) each person in turn describes something that they are looking forward to;
    (b) each person in turn describes his house, car or some other fairly 'neutral' object.

5. The facilitator self-evaluates her own performance by describing the short-comings and strengths of her facilitation to the group.
6. The facilitator invites peer evaluation by asking for feedback from the group on her performance. It is helpful if group members first say what they *did not like* about her facilitation and then what they *liked* about it.

Notes

It is recommended that the group facilitator who wishes to develop a wide range of cathartic skills considers undergoing specific training in them. Training courses in managing other people's emotions are often offered by colleges, polytechnics and university departments, particularly those with an interest in humanistic psychology and 'growth' work.

Exercise 58

Aim of the exercise: To exercise a non-cathartic style of group facilitation.
Group size: Any number from 6 to 20.
Time required: About 1 hour.
Materials and/or environment required: A large, comfortable room and a circle of straight-backed chairs.

Process

1. The facilitator either decides on a topic for discussion or negotiates a topic with the group.
2. During the discussion that follows, the facilitator purposely avoids issues that are emotionally charged and if emotional issues do arise, deflects them by moving the discussion onto a lighter level.
3. After half an hour the facilitator draws the discussion to a close and summarizes the content and process of the discussion as necessary.
4. The facilitator self-evaluates his own performance by describing the short-comings and strengths of his facilitation to the group.
5. The facilitator invites peer evaluation by asking for feedback from the group on his performance. It is helpful if group members first say what they *did not like* about his facilitation and then what they *liked* about it.

Notes

The skill of moving between levels of emotion in group work is an important one. Even when a contract has been drawn up with a particular group that allows the expression of emotion, it is important the facilitator does not 'hound' the group or overstate the need for emotional release. The facilitator who can use a light approach, even with heavyweight topics, is likely to be more successful that the one who is always earnest and meaningful in her approach. Paradoxically, the light approach can often allow for a far greater expression of emotion than can the 'earnest' approach.

Aim of the exercise: To exercise a structuring style of group facilitation.
Group size: Any number from 6 to 20.
Time required: Between 1 and 2 hours.
Materials and/or environment required: A large, comfortable room and a circle of straight-backed chairs.

Process

1. The facilitator introduces and explains the rules of a structured exercise or activity to the group. One from the earlier part of this chapter may be used. Others are described by Kagan, Evans and Kay (1986).
2. The group undertakes the exercise and the facilitator pays close attention to giving clear instructions and keeps a close eye on timing.
3. The facilitator invites the group to reconvene after the exercise and asks each member of the group to complete the following two sentences:
   (a) 'What I liked least about this exercise was ...';
   (b) 'What I liked most about this exercise was ...'.
3. The facilitator self-evaluates her own performance by describing the shortcomings and strengths of her facilitation to the group.
4. The facilitator invites peer evaluation by asking for feedback from the group on her performance. It is helpful if group members first say what they *did not like* about her facilitation and then what they *liked* about it.

Notes

It has been noted above that it is often a good idea to *start* a series of group meetings with plenty of structure. Too little can make the meetings seem aimless. Structure can easily be dropped as the group develops a sense of identity. On the other hand, it is often difficult to *introduce* structure if it has not been there previously.

Aim of the exercise: To exercise an unstructuring style of group facilitation.
Group size: Any number from 6 to 20.
Time required: About 1 hour.
Materials and/or environment required: A large, comfortable room and a circle of straight-backed chairs.

Process

1. The facilitator invites suggestions from the group as to any exercises, games etc. that the group would like to undertake.
2. The facilitator, may, as required, invite a member of the group to take over group facilitation for the exercise.
3. Alternatively, the facilitator helps the group to undertake the exercise but remains an almost equal member of the group and does not try to impose any structure on what is happening.
4. After the activity has been completed, the facilitator self-evaluates his own performance by describing the shortcomings and strengths of his facilitation to the group.
5. The facilitator invites peer evaluation by asking for feedback from the group on his performance. It is helpful if group members first say what they *did not like* about his facilitation and then what they *liked* about it.

Exercise 61

Aim of the exercise: To explore lack of structure in a group setting.
Group size: Any number from 6 to 20.
Time required: About $1\frac{1}{2}$ hours.
Materials and/or environment required: A large, comfortable room and a circle of straight-backed chairs.

Process

1. The facilitator walks into the group, sits down and remains silent for the duration of an hour. She allows the group to unfold (or not) as it will.
2. At the end of the hour she declares the exercise complete and invokes a discussion on the experience.
3. The facilitator self-evaluates her own performance by describing the shortcomings and strengths of her facilitation to the group.
4. The facilitator invites peer evaluation by asking for feedback from the group on her performance. It is helpful if group members first say what they *did not like* about her facilitation and then what they *liked* about it.

Notes

This is the extreme example of an unstructuring approach. A similar approach, from a therapeutic point of view, is described by Bion (1961), in his classic book on running groups. Often, the following stages may be observed with this activity:

(a) the group is confused and sometimes amused by what is happening;
(b) several, usually abortive attempts are made to take over leadership and begin an activity;
(c) the group gets angry with the facilitator for not carrying out her 'proper' role;
(d) the group ignores the facilitator and attempts to carry on as though she were not there.

This format requires a certain bravery on the part of the facilitator (and on the part of the group!) but it can be a useful way of exploring issues of dependency and independence.

Exercise 62

Aim of the exercise: To exercise a disclosing style of group facilitation.
Group size: Any number from 6 to 20.
Time required: About 1 hour.
Materials and/or environment required: A large, comfortable room and a circle of straight-backed chairs.

Process

1. The facilitator shares a story, anecdote or persona experience with the group and develops a discussion based on it.
2. During the discussion the facilitator shares his immediate and/or past experiences with group members.
3. After three-quarters of an hour, the facilitator sums up the content and process of the group as required, or invites the group members to do so.
4. The facilitator self-evaluates his own performance by describing the shortcomings and strengths of his facilitation to the group.
5. The facilitator invites peer evaluation by asking for feedback from the group on his performance. It is helpful if group members first say what they *did not like* about his facilitation and then what they *liked* about it.

Exercise 63

Aim of the exercise: To exercise a non-disclosing style of group leadership.
Group size: Any number from 6 to 20.
Time required: About 1 hour.
Materials and/or environment required: A large, comfortable room and a circle of straight-backed chairs.

Process

1. The facilitator invites stories, anecdotes or experiences from the group and develops a discussion around them.
2. During the discussion that follows the facilitator encourages the sharing of experiences by members of the group but at no point discloses her own feelings or thoughts. She deflects any direct questions from group members.
3. After half an hour, the facilitator draws the discussion to a close and sums up the content and process of the activity as required.
4. The facilitator self-evaluates her own performance by describing the shortcomings and strengths of her facilitation to the group.

5. The facilitator invites peer evaluation by asking for feedback from the group on her performance. It is helpful if group members first say what they *did not like* about her facilitation and then what they *liked* about it.

Notes

Disclosure begets disclosure (Jourard, 1964). The disclosing facilitator can often encourage the group to talk more freely and easily once they realize that she is also prepared to give of herself. On the other hand, it is easy to *over disclose*. The facilitator who discloses too much, too quickly is likely to alienate herself from the group who think: 'Am *I* going to have to reveal *myself* in this way?' Judging levels of disclosure is a fairly precise business.

Recording and evaluating group work

It is often helpful to know how a group is changing as it works together. One very simple format for checking, verbally, on progress in the group is to ask at the end of a session or a day for the group to work through two 'rounds'. During the first round, each person in turn completes the sentence: 'What I liked least about this session was . . .'. When everybody has completed the statement, a second round is completed using the sentence: 'What I liked most about this session was . . .'. This offers a quick and subjective method of evaluation. Another approach is to hold a short 'unfinished business' session at the end of each day. Ten minutes is left at the end in which anyone is free to say anything, positive or negative about the day. They are free to surface any doubts, annoyances, pleasant experiences – anything. They may also want to say something to another member of the group that up to that point they had only been thinking. The idea behind this 'air clearing' activity is that it is probably as well to verbalize some of these thoughts and feelings that are just below the surface rather than to carry them out of the group. During the unfinished business session, the facilitator does not respond to the statements that are made other than by accepting them.

Another, more permanent method of charting progress is through the use of a visual device such as the one developed out of Cox's (1978) work (Figure 7.7). Each circle represents one of the group members. Each circle can be divided up in any way that the facilitator finds useful and each segment of the circle can then be used to record notes about each member of the group. A fresh record sheet is kept for each meeting of the group and the collected sheets serves as an evaluation device.

An alternative to this is that the circles are drawn on a large sheet of paper and group members record their feelings and thoughts at the end of each session. The sheets are then kept for display whilst subsequent meetings are in progress.

Other methods of assessment, both objective and subjective, may be used to chart educational progress if the focus of the group is mainly an

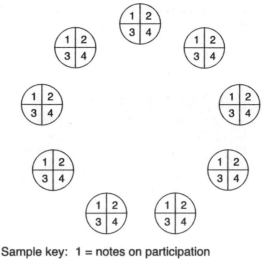

Sample key: 1 = notes on participation
2 = mood
3 = attitude toward others in the group
4 = other notes

Figure 7.7   A format for recording group progress (after Cox, 1978)

educational or training one. Neil Kenworthy and Peter Nicklin offer an excellent review of up-to-date assessment methods (Kenworthy and Nicklin, 1989).

Through the series of exercises in group membership and group facilitation described in this chapter, skills can be developed that may be carried over into any nursing situation. That they *are* carried over is a fundamental issue. Clearly, any amount of group work in the context of nursing is of little value if it does not lead to a positive change in nursing practice. Sometimes the transfer of learning takes place at a subtle level: the nurse modifies her attitudes or takes more notice of what she does and says. Sometimes the change is quite clear and nursing students begin to set up groups and run them effectively. It is important, though, that constant reference to nursing is made during training sessions that incorporate the exercises in this chapter.

Finally, an outline programme for a workshop on group facilitation skills is offered that can be adapted for use in any nurse education or training course.

A programme for group facilitation training

Introductions

1. The group facilitator introduces the aims of the workshop and outlines domestic arrangements: meal breaks and tea and coffee breaks.
2. The facilitator invites the group members to introduce themselves using the approach outlined in this book. Icebreakers can also be used as required.

3. The facilitator discusses the aims of the workshop and introduces the two principles:
   (a) the voluntary principle: that everyone is free to take part in activities or to sit out of them as they see fit;
   (b) the proposal clause: that group members should take responsibility for suggesting that the group either spends more time on a certain section of the workshop or that things are speeded up.

Theory input

1. The facilitator offers a short theory input on group theory and group dynamics.
2. The group undertake one or two group membership exercises (e.g. Exercises 30–50 from this book).
3. The facilitator introduces the concept of Dimensions of Facilitator Styles and discusses these with the group.

Experiential learning activities

1. Individual members of the group take turns in leading the group by working with different styles of group facilitation (Exercises 51–63 in this book).
2. Volunteers then lead the group for longer periods (between 1 and 2 hours using EITHER one particular style OR using an eclectic style incorporating many different aspects of the dimensions of facilitator styles. The latter choice is not a good one early on in a course as it is often difficult for group members (and the facilitator) to determine what style is being used at any given time.
3. The volunteers from (2) above self-evaluate their facilitation skills in front of the group and invite feedback from the group and from the facilitator of the workshop.

Evaluation and application

1. A final plenary session is held to discuss the application of the new skills to the clinical or community setting.
2. The facilitator leads a evaluation session and closes the workshop.

This format can be adapted for use as a 1- or 2-day workshop, a week-long workshop or as a series of study days.

Formal evaluation

Most educational and training organizations are now required to evaluate their courses more formally as part of an audit trail. Figure 7.8 is an example of a questionnaire that can be used at the end of an experiential workshop – in this case, on counselling. The questionnaire can easily be adapted to suit other sorts of workshops, including those involving group work.

Course participants are given photocopies of the questionnaire on the last day of the workshop and asked to fill them in before they leave. They can, of course, be completed anonymously but it is important to make sure that every participant hands in a completed questionnaire.

Newtown College of Health and Science

Counselling Skills Workshop

Workshop Evaluation Form

We are committed to maintaining and strengthening the quality of the courses that we offer to participants. I would be grateful if you would take a few minutes to complete this form and to add any comments that you may have about how the Counselling Workshop might be improved. Your comments will be discussed by the teaching staff and reported to the Board of Health Care Studies.

Andrew Davies
Workshop leader

1. I feel that the aims of the workshop have been achieved

Strongly agree	Agree	Don't know	Disagree	Strongly disagree
1 ✓	2	3	4	5

Comments
I appreciated the fact that we were invited to identify some of our *own* aims for the workshop
....

2. Varied teaching and learning methods have been used throughout the workshop

Strongly agree	Agree	Don't know	Disagree	Strongly disagree
1	2 ✓	3	4	5

Comments
I enjoyed the exercises in pairs
....

3. Most students have taken an active part in the workshop

Strongly agree	Agree	Don't know	Disagree	Strongly disagree
1 ✓	2	3	4	5

Comments
Two participants sometimes dominated the group
....

4. The quality of the teaching on this course was high

Strongly agree	Agree	Don't know	Disagree	Strongly disagree
1	2	3 ✓	4	5

Comments
I have little experience - difficult to judge
....

Workshop Evalualtion Form *(cont)*

5. The content of this workshop will help me in my work

Strongly agree	Agree	Don't know	Disagree	Strongly disagree
1	2	3	4 ✓	5

Comments
I'm not sure that I will, automatically, be able to apply this
....

6. The lecture room/teaching accommodation was satisfactory

Strongly agree	Agree	Don't know	Disagree	Strongly disagree
1 ✓	2	3	4	5

Comments
....

7. Access to teaching accommodation was good and I was able to get to the sessions on time

Strongly agree	Agree	Don't know	Disagree	Strongly disagree
1 ✓	2	3	4	5

Comments
....

8. Generally, the workshop seems well organized

Strongly agree	Agree	Don't know	Disagree	Strongly disagree
1 ✓	2	3	4	5

Comments
I would have liked some more on breaking bad news but, generally, it was very interesting and useful
....

9. Please identify, below, any issues that you feel need to be addressed in order to improve the quality of the counselling workshop

As a manager in the health service, I would like to have had more input on how to deal with difficult situations. The general counselling training, though, was excellent. I enjoyed the course and learned a lot from it. The exercises in pairs were particularly useful and I think I learned a lot about myself and about how bossy I can be, sometimes! There probably needs to be more *breaks* in the course

Thank you for your time,
Andrew Davies,
Workshop leader

Figure 7.8   Example of counselling workshop evaluation form

Participants simply tick the box after each question that most nearly matches their response to the item. After each item, there is space for more general comments.

Participants should be reminded to respond to every item and to tick only one box against each item. They should be instructed, too, that their responses will be treated in confidence and will help in the planning of future courses. This final point must, of course, be true – there is little point in asking for formal course feedback if the information obtained is not *used*. It is vital that the workshop leader collates the information gained from these questionnaires and uses it to guide future curriculum and workshop planning.

Processing the evaluation questionnaire

Having asked participants to complete the questionnaire, the next stage is to organize the data from them in ways that will make reading the 'results' possible. The first stage is to undertake frequency counts of the numbers of responses to each option following each of the items. This is easily achieved with a spreadsheet.

The first stage is to collate the findings from the questionnaire items into a table in a spreadsheet, as illustrated in Figure 7.9.

The next stage is to ask the spreadsheet to run frequency counts for each column of the chart. When instructed this way, the spreadsheet program will compute how many '1's, '2's, '3's, '4's and '5's there were for each item and will sort these into what the spreadsheet calls 'bins'. From this process, it will be possible to see at a glance how the workshop participants scored their questionnaires – as in Figure 7.10.

If participants offer 'comments' under the questionnaire items, these can be brought together under a series of headings, as in the example in Figure 7.11. For larger workshops and larger groups of participants, there are computer programs such as The Ethnograph, PinPoint and NUD.IST that can be used for this purpose. For small groups, it is probably easiest to collate the comments by hand as not everyone will put comments under each of the items and many people will, perhaps, not offer comments at all.

Recommended reading

Bertcher, H.J. and Maple, F. (1996) *Creating Groups*, 2nd edn. London, Sage.

Burnard, P. (1996) *Acquiring Interpersonal Skills – A Handbook of Experiential Learning for Health Professionals*, 2nd edn. Cheltenham, Nelson-Thornes.

Burnard, P. (1997) *Effective Communication Skills for Health Professionals*, 2nd edn. Cheltenham, Nelson-Thornes.

Kagan, C. and Evans, J. (1994) *Professional Interpersonal Skills for Nurses*, 2nd edn. Cheltenham, Nelson-Thornes.

Kurtz, L.F. (1997) *Self-Help and Support Groups: A Handbook for Practitioners*. London, Sage.

Wetherell, M. (ed.) (1996) *Identities, Groups and Social Issues*. London, Sage.

	Quest1	Quest2	Quest3	Quest4	Quest5	Quest6	Quest7	Quest8
Participant 1	1	2	1	3	4	1	1	1
Participant 2	2	1	2	1	1	1	2	2
Participant 3	2	2	2	3	3	3	4	5
Participant 4	1	2	2	1	1	2	3	2
Participant 5	1	1	1	1	1	1	2	1
Participant 6	2	1	2	3	2	1	3	4
Participant 7	4	2	1	1	2	3	4	1
Participant 8	1	4	2	2	1	2	1	1
Participant 9	5	4	3	3	5	3	5	5
Participant 10	3	1	1	3	1	2	1	1

Figure 7.9   Spreadsheet display of questionnaire results

Item 1: I feel that the aims of the workshop have been achieved ($n = 10$)

Strongly agreed	4
Agreed	3
Didn't know	1
Disagreed	1
Strongly disagreed	1

Figure 7.10   Displayed result of a frequency count analysis

Comments on Item 1: I feel that the aims of the workshop have been achieved

'I appreciated the fact that we were invited to identify some of our *own* aims for the workshop.'

'Too much time was spent in discussing the aims of the course. I felt we could have moved on a bit quicker.'

'The aims session was useful. It helped me to think about what we were doing.'

'The group was allowed to argue and debate too long. This seemed like a waste of time to me.'

'The main aims were clearly stated in the handout at the beginning of the workshop.'

Figure 7.11   Grouping of comments on an item from the questionnaire

Appendix 1:
Topics for Pairs Activities

The pairs format described in Chapter 6 is a particularly flexible one for use in the experiential learning mode. The following questions are ones that can be used in that format to explore aspects of self-awareness and interpersonal skills.

These questions can be used in the following way. Members of a learning group pair off and are nominated 'A' and 'B'. A then poses the particular question and listens to B's answer. A then *repeats* the question after two further intervals, so that B can fully explore the question. The activity is not a conversation and A's only task is to listen. After 10 minutes, roles are reversed and B poses the question to A, three times over a period of 10 minutes. When both partners have had their turns, a plenary session is convened.

- Who are you? (This is an alarmingly straightforward question that can usefully be explored at different times during a group's life.)
- What are the personal qualities that make *you* an effective nurse (or counsellor)?
- What do you need to do to become a more effective nurse (or counsellor)?
- How do you look after yourself?
- How do you demonstrate care for others?
- What do you need to do to enhance your care for others?
- How do you feel about yourself?
- What are your best qualities?
- What do others think and feel about you?
- If you had to change some of your personal characteristics, which ones would you change?
- If you had to live in another period in history, which one would you live in ... can you expand on the topic?
- What are your most important beliefs about yourself/your work/your personal life/your relationships?
- What do you need to do to enhance your relationships with others?
- What (if any) spiritual beliefs do you have?
- What have been the most important things that you have learned?
- What would you change about nursing?
- What would you change about other people?
- What sorts of things would you change about society?
- If you were to do something other than nursing, what would it be ... can you expand ...?

- In what ways has nursing changed you?
- What sorts of situations would you find *most difficult* in counselling?
- What sorts of situations would you find *most difficult* in running groups?
- What do you need to do to enhance your facilitation skills?

Appendix 2:
Topics for Group Activities

Chapter 5 describes a range of group activities for use in exploring group membership and group facilitation. The following topics are ones that can be used instead of the suggested ones or as supplementary topics.

- Nurse education and nursing
- Running groups
- Being a nurse counsellor
- Being a group facilitator
- Nursing models and nursing theory
- The theory–practice gap in nursing
- Why do we need self-awareness?
- Stress and nursing
- Problems in running groups
- Problems in being a group member
- Dealing with aggression
- Coping with anxiety
- Our relationships with each other in this group
- The pros and cons of group activities
- How we've changed as a group
- What we would like to change about the people in this group
- How we are the same as each other and how we differ
- Management and education in nursing
- Difficult patients
- How we could become more assertive
- What we do with our anger
- How we deal with stress
- Socialization into nursing
- How we could be different
- Our beliefs as a group
- What would happen to the group if various members left
- Interpersonal skills training in nursing
- Coping with bereavement

References

Alberti, R.E. and Emmons, M.L. (1982) *Your Perfect Right: A Guide to Assertive Living*, 4th edn. San Luis, Impact Publishers.

Alexander, F.M. (1969) *Resurrection of the Body*. New York, University Books.

Argyle, M. (1975) *The Psychology of Interpersonal Behaviour*. Harmondsworth, Penguin.

Arnold, E. and Boggs, K. (1989) *Interpersonal Relationships: Professional Communication Skills for Nurses*. Philadelphia, Saunders.

Atkins, S. and Murphy, K. (1993) Reflection: a review of the literature. *Journal of Advanced Nursing*, 18: 1188–92.

Bandler, R. and Grinder, J. (1975) *The Structure of Magic*, vol. 1: *A Book about Language and Therapy*. California, Science and Behaviour Books.

Bannister, D. and Fransella, F. (1986) *Inquiring Man: The Psychology of Personal Constructs*, 3rd edn. London, Croom Helm.

Baruth, L.G. (1987) *An Introduction to the Counselling Profession*. Englewood Cliffs, NJ, Prentice Hall.

Bateson, C.D. and Coke, J.S. (1981) Empathy: a source of altruistic motivation for helping? In J.P. Rushton and R.M. Sorventino, *Altruism and Helping Behavior: Social, Personality and Developmental Perspectives*. Hillsdale, NJ, Lawrence Erlbaum Associates.

Beder, H. (1987) Dominant paradigms, adult education and social justice. *Adult Education Quarterly*, 2: 105–13.

Bedi, N., Chilvers, C., Churchill, R. et al. (2000) Assessing effectiveness of treatment of depression in primary care: partially randomised preference trial. *British Journal of Psychiatry*, 177: 312–18.

Belkin, G.S. (1984) *Introduction to Counselling*. Dubuque, IO, Brown.

Bion, W. (1961) *Experiences in Groups*. London, Tavistock.

Blake, R.R. and Mouton, J.S. (1976) *Consultation*. New York, Addison Wesley.

Bond, M. (1986) *Stress and Self-Awareness: A Guide for Nurses*. London, Heinemann.

Bond, M. (1987) *Being Assertive: A Distance Learning Pack for Nurses*. London, Distance Learning Centre, South Bank Polytechnic.

Bond, M. and Kilty, J. (1982) *Practical Methods of Coping With Stress*. Guildford, Human Potential Research Project, University of Surrey.

Bond, S. and Rhodes, T. (1990) HIV infection and community midwives: experience and practice. *Midwifery*, 6: 33–40.

Bond, S., Rhodes, T., Philips, P., Fox, C. and Bond, J. (1990) HIV infection and AIDS in England: the experience, knowledge and intentions of community nursing staff. *Journal of Advanced Nursing*, 15: 249–55.

Boore, J. (1978) *A Prescription for Recovery*. London, RCN.

Boud, D. (ed.) (1981) *Developing Student Autonomy in Learning.* London, Kogan Page.

Boud, D. (1989) The role of self assessment in student grading, in *Assessment and Evaluation in Higher Education* Vol. 14 no. 1, pp. 20–30.

Boud, D. and Pascoe, J. (1978) *Experiential Learning: Developments in Australian Post-secondary Education.* Sydney, Australian Consortium on Experiential Learning.

Bower, P., Byford, S., Sibbald, B. *et al.* (2000) Randomised controlled trial of non-directive counselling, cognitive-behaviour therapy and usual GP care for patients with depression. II: Cost effectiveness. *British Medical Journal*, 321: 1389–92.

Boyd, E.M. and Fales, A.W. (1983) Reflective learning: key to learning from experience. *Journal of Humanistic Psychology*, 23 (2): 99–117.

Briggs, K. (1992) Breaking the silence. *Nursing Times*, 88 (40): 50–1.

Brookfield, S.D. (1987) *Developing Critical Thinkers: Challenging Adults to Explore Alternative Ways of Thinking and Acting.* Milton Keynes, Open University Press.

Brookfield, S.D. (1986) *Understanding and Facilitating Adult Learning.* Milton Keynes, Open University Press.

Brown, R. (1965) *Social Psychology.* London, Collier Macmillan.

Brown, S.D. and Lent, R.W. (eds) (1984) *Handbook of Counselling Psychology.* Chichester.

Buber, M. (1958) *I and Thou.* New York, Scribener.

Buber, M. (1965) *The Knowledge of Man.* New York, Harper and Row.

Bugental, E. and Bugental, J. (1984) Dispiritedness – a new perspective on a familiar state. *Journal of Humanistic Psychology*, 24 (1): 49–67.

Burkhardt, M. and Nagai-Jacobson, M. (1985) Dealing with spiritual concerns of clients in the community. *Journal of Community Health Nursing*, 2 (4): 191–8.

Burnard, P. (1989a) *Counselling Skills for Health Professionals.* London, Chapman and Hall.

Burnard, P. (1989b) *Teaching Interpersonal Skills: A Handbook of Experiential Learning for Health Professionals.* London, Chapman and Hall.

Burnard, P. (1989c) Exploring nurse educators' views of experiential learning. *Nurse Education Today*, 9: 39–45.

Burnard, P. (1991) *Experiential Learning in Action.* Aldershot, Avebury.

Burnard, P. and Morrison, P. (1988) Nurses' perceptions of their interpersonal skills: a descriptive study using six category intervention analysis. *Nurse Education Today*, 8: 266–72.

Burnard, P. and Morrison, P. (1992) *Self-Disclosure: A Contemporary Analysis.* Avebury, Aldershot.

Campbell, A. (1984) *Moderated Love.* London, SPCK.

Canfield, J. and Wells, H.C. (1976) *100 Ways to Enhance Self Concept in the Classroom.* Englewood Cliffs, NJ, Prentice Hall.

Chilvers, C., Dewey, M., Fielding, K. *et al.* (2001) Antidepressant drugs and generic counselling for treatment of major depression in primary care: randomised trial with patient preference arms. *British Medical Journal*, 322: 775.

Clarke, B. and Feltham, W. (1990) Facilitating peer group teaching within nurse education, *Nurse Education Today*, 10: 54–7.

Claxton, G. (1984) *Live and Learn: An Introduction to the Psychology of Growth and Change in Everyday Life.* London, Harper and Row.

Conrad, J. (1911) *Under Western Eyes.* Harmondsworth, Penguin.

Cook, R. (1992) Uninhibited introductions. *Nursing Standard*, 17 (7): 46.

Cowan, J. and Garry, A. (1986) *Learning from Experience*. London, Further Education Unit.

Cox, M. (1978) *Structuring the Therapeutic Process*. London, Pergamon.

Cullinan, R. (1991) Health visitor intervention in postnatal depression. *Health Visitor*, 64 (12): 412–13.

Daniel, C. (1992) Counselling sexual abuse survivors, *Nursing Standard*, 6 (46): 28–31.

Devine, E.C. and Cook, T.D. (1983) A meta-analytical analysis of effects of psychoeducational interventions on length of postsurgical hospital stay. *Nursing Research*, 32 (5): 267–74.

Dewey, J. (1933) *How We Think*. Boston, D.C. Heath.

Dewey, J. (1958) *Experience and Nature*. New York, Dover.

Dewey, J. (1966) *Democracy and Education*. New York, The Free Press/Macmillan.

Dewey, J. (1971) *Experience and Education*. New York, Collier Macmillan.

Egan, G. (1986) *The Skilled Helper*. Monterey, CA, Brooks Cole.

Eliot, T.S. (1930/1963) 'Ash-Wednesday', in *Collected Poems* 1909–1962. London, Faber, p. 96.

Ellerhorst-Ryan, J. (1985) Selecting an instrument to measure spiritual distress, *Oncology Nursing Forum*, 12 (2): 93–9.

Ellis, D. (1980) Whatever happened to the spiritual dimension?, *Canadian Nurse*, 76 (2): 42–3.

Ellis, R. and Whittington, D. (1981) *A Guide to Social Skills Training*. London, Croom Helm.

Engstrom, B. (1984) The patients need for information during hospital stay, *International Journal of Nursing Studies*, 21: 113–30.

Evans, N. (1985) *Post-Education Society: Recognizing Adults as Learners*. London, Croom Helm.

Evans, N. (1992) *Experiential Learning*. London, Routledge.

Feldenkrais, M. (1972) *Awareness Through Movement*. New York, Harper and Row.

Field, P.A. and Morse, J.M. (1985) *Nursing Research: The Application of Qualitative Approaches*. London, Croom Helm.

Freire, P. (1970) *Cultural Action for Freedom*. Harmondsworth, Penguin.

Freire, P. (1972) *Pedagogy of the Oppressed*. Harmondsworth, Penguin.

Freire, P. (1974) *Education for Critical Consciousness*. Continuum, New York.

Freire, P. (1985) *The Politics of Education*. South Hadley, MA, Bergin and Garvey.

Freire, P. (1986) Keynote Address. Presented at Workshop on Worker Education, City College of New York Center for Worker Education, New York, 8 February.

Friedli, K., King, M. and Lloyd M. *et al.* (1997) Randomised controlled assessment of non-directive psychotherapy versus routine general-practitioner care. *Lancet*, 350: 1662–5.

Fromm, E. (1965) *Fear of Freedom*. London: Routledge.

Fromm, E. (1975) *The Art of Loving*. London, Allen and Unwin.

Fromm, E. (1979) *To Have or To Be?* London, Abacus.

Gale, D. (1989) Moreno's approach to humanistic psychology: self and society. *European Journal of Humanistic Psychology*, 17 (7): 9–14.

Garnets, L., Hancock, K.A., Cochran, S.D., Goodchild, J. and Peplau, L.A. (1991) Issues in psychotherapy with lesbians and gay men. *American Psychologist*, 46 (9): 964–72.

Geertz, C. (1966) *Anthropological Approaches to Religion*. London, Tavistock.

Geller, L. (1984) Another look at self-actualisation. *Journal of Humanistic Psychology*, 24 (2): 93–106.

Gilbert, N. (1993) *Researching Social Life*. London, Sage.

Goble, J. (1990) Psychodrama takes central stage. *Nursing Times*, 86 (28): 34–5.

Granstrom, S. (1985) Spiritual nursing care for oncology patients. *Topics in Clinical Nursing*, 7 (1): 35–45.

Gray, H. (1986) Experiential learning with adults: self and society. *European Journal of Humanistic Psychology*, 4 (6): 282–6.

Hanscombe, G.E. and Humphries, M. (1987) *Heterosexuality*. GMP Publishers, London.

Hargie, O., Saunders, C. and Dickson, D. (1987) *Social Skills in Interpersonal Communication*. London, Croom Helm.

Hargie, O., Saunders, C. and Dickson, D. (1994) *Social Skills in Interpersonal Communication*, 3rd edn. London, Routledge.

Harvey, I., Nelson, S., Lyons, R. *et al.* (1988) Randomized controlled trial and economic evaluation of counselling in primary care. *British Journal of General Practice*, 48: 1043–8.

Hayward, J. (1975) *Information: A Prescription Against Pain*. London, RCN.

Hazzard, A. (1995) Measuring outcome in counselling: a brief exploration of the issues. *British Journal of General Practice*, 45: 118–19.

Hemmings, A. (1997) Counselling in primary care: a randomised controlled trial. *Patient Education and Counselling*, 32: 219–30.

Henderson, P. and Foster, G. (1991) *Groupwork*. Cambridge, The National Extension College.

Heron, J. (1970) *The Phenomenology of the Gaze*. Guildford, Human Potential Research Project, University of Surrey.

Heron, J. (1973) *Experiential Training Techniques*. Guildford, Human Potential Research Project, University of Surrey.

Heron, J. (1974) Open Letter to Harvey Jackins: self and society. *European Journal of Humanistic Psychology*, No. 5.

Heron, J. (1977a) *Catharsis in Human Development*. Guildford, Human Potential Research Project, University of Surrey.

Heron, J. (1977b) *Behaviour Analysis in Education and Training*. Guildford, Human Potential Research Project, University of Surrey.

Heron, J. (1978) *Co-Counselling Teacher's Manual*. Guildford, Human Potential Research Project, University of Surrey.

Heron, J. (1981) Philosophical basis for a new paradigm. In P. Reason and J. Rowan (eds), *Human Inquiry: A Sourcebook of New Paradigm Research*. Chichester, Wiley.

Heron, J. (1986) *Six Category Intervention Analysis*, 2nd edn. Guildford, Human Potential Research Project, University of Surrey.

Heron, J. (1989a) *Six Category Intervention Analysis*, 3rd edn. Guildford, Human Potential Resource Group, University of Surrey.

Heron, J. (1989b) *A Handbook of Facilitator Style*. London, Kogan Page.

Heron, J. and Reason, P. (1981) *Co-Counselling: An Experiential Inquiry I*. Guildford, Human Potential Resource Group, University of Surrey.

Heron, J. and Reason, P. (1982) *Co-Counselling: An Experiential Inquiry II*. Guildford, University of Surrey, Human Potential Resource Group.

Hopkinson, C. (1994) Warm-up exercises: can learning be fun? *Nursing Standard*, 8 (37): 30–4.

Hopper, E. (1991) Shattered dreams. *Nursing Standard*, 6 (4): 20–1.

Illich, I. (1973) *Deschooling Society*. Harmondsworth, Penguin.

Jackins, H. (1965) *The Human Side of Human Beings*. Seattle, Rational Island Publishers.

Jackins, H. (1970) *Fundamentals of Co-counselling Manual*. Seattle, Rational Island Publishers.

Jackins, H. (1983) *The Reclaiming of Power*. Seattle, Rational Island Publishers.

Jarvis, P. (1983) *The Theory and Practice of Adult and Continuing Education*. London, Croom Helm.

Jarvis, P. (1984) *The Sociology of Adult and Continuing Education*. London, Croom Helm.

Jarvis, P. (1992) Reflective practice and nursing. *Nurse Education Today*, 12: 174–81.

Jennings, S. (1992) A lifeline offering support: nurses role in fertility counselling. *Professional Nurse*, May, pp. 539–42.

Johns, C. (1993a) On becoming effective in taking ethical action. *Journal of Clinical Nursing*, 2: 307–12.

Johns, C. (1993b) Professional supervision. *Journal of Nursing Management*, 1: 9–18.

Johnson, A.W. and Nadirshaw, Z. (1993) Good practice in transcultural counselling: an Asian perspective. *British Journal of Guidance and Counselling*, 21 (1): 20–9.

Jones, A. (1990a) Looking death in the face. *Nursing Times*, 86 (40): 50–2.

Jones, A. (1990b) Empathy in the counselling process. *Nursing Standard*, 4 (44): 53–5.

Jones, A. (1990c) All you ever wanted to know about counselling, *Nursing Times*, 86 (12): 55–8.

Jones, K. (1991) *Icebreakers: A Sourcebook of Games, Exercises and Simulations*. London, Kogan Page.

Jourard, S. (1959) Self-disclosure and other-cathexis. *Journal of Abnormal and Social Psychology*, 59: 528–31.

Jourard, S. (1961) Self disclosure in British and American college females. *Journal of Social Psychology*, 54: 315–20.

Jourard, S. (1964) *The Transparent Self*. New York, Van Nostrand.

Jourard, S. (1971) *Self-Disclosure, an Experimental Analysis of the Transparent Self*. New York, Wiley.

Jung, C.G. (1978) *Man and His Symbols*. London, Picador.

Jung, C.G. (1938/1961) Psychology and religion. In *Collected Works*, Vol. 2. London, Routledge and Kegan Paul.

Kagan, C. (ed.) (1985) *Interpersonal Skills in Nursing: Research and Applications*. London, Croom Helm.

Kagan, C., Evans, J. and Kay, B. (1986) *A Manual of Interpersonal Skills for Nurses: An Experiential Approach*. London, Harper and Row.

Kalisch, B.J. (1971) Strategies for developing nurse empathy. *Nurse Education*, 19 (11): 714–17.

Kant, I. (1985) *Fundamental Principles of the Metaphysics of Morals*. New York, Library of Liberal Arts.

Kelly, G.A. (1955) *The Psychology of Interpersonal Constructs*, Vols 1 and 2. New York, Norton.

Kemmis S. (1985) Action research and the politics of reflection. In D. Boud (ed.), *Reflection: Turning Experience into Learning*. New York, Nichols, pp. 139–62.

Kenworthy, N. and Nicklin, P. (1989) *Teaching and Assessing in Nursing Practice: An Experiential Approach*. London, Scutari.

Kilty, J. (1982) *Experiential Learning*. Guildford, Human Potential Research Project, University of Surrey.

Kirschenbaum, H. (1979) *On Becoming Carl Rogers*. New York, Dell.

Knowles, M. (1975) *Self-Directed Learning*. New York, Cambridge Books.

Knowles, M. (1978) *The Adult Learner: A Neglected Species*, 2nd edn. Houston, TX, Gulf.

Knowles, M. (1980) *The Modern Theory and Practice of Adult Education*. Chicago, Follett.

Knowles, M. (1984) *Andragogy in Action: Applying Modern Principles of Adult Learning*. San Francisco, Jossey Bass.

Koberg, D. and Bagnall, D. (1981) *The Revised All New Universal Traveler: A Soft-Systems Guide to Creativity and Problem Solving and the Process of Reaching Goals*. Los Altos, CA, Kaufmann.

Kolb, D. (1984) *Experiential Learning*. Englewood Cliffs, NJ, Prentice Hall.

Kwast, B.E. (1992) Abortion: its contribution to maternal mortality, *Midwifery*, 8: 8–11.

Labun, E. (1988) Spiritual care, an element in nursing care planning. *Journal of Advanced Nursing*, 13: 314–20.

Lai, P., Hubbling, D. and Persaud R. (1998) Non-directive counselling versus routine general practitioner care (letter). *Lancet*, 351: 750.

Laing, R.D. (1959) *The Divided Self*. Harmondsworth, Penguin.

Landrine, H. (1992) Clinical implications of cultural differences: the referential vs the indexical self. *Clinical Psychology Review*, 12: 401–15.

Lane, J. (1987) The care of the human spirit. *Journal of Professional Nursing*, 3 (6): 332–7.

Lawrence, Brother (1981) *The Practice of the Presence of God*. Sevenoaks, Hodder and Stoughton.

Lee, H. (1960) *To Kill a Mockingbird*. London, Heinemann.

Lindell, M. and Olsson, H. (1991) Can combined oral contraceptives be made more effective by means of a nursing care model? *Journal of Advanced Nursing*, 16: 475–9.

Lindeman, E. (1956) The democratic man. In Gessner, R. (ed.), *Selected Writings*. Boston, MA, Beacon Press.

Liss, J. (1974) *Free to Feel*. London, Wildwood House.

LoBiondo-Wood, G. and Haber, J. (1994) *Nursing Research: Methods, Critical Appraisal and Utilization*, 3rd edn. St Louis, Mosby.

Lowen, A. (1967) *The Betrayal of the Body*. New York, Macmillan.

Luft, J. (1969) *Of Human Interaction: The Johari Model*. Palo Alto, CA, Mayfield.

Lugton, J. (1989) Making plans. *Nursing Times*, 18 (10): 44–5.

Lyte, V.J. and Thompson, I.G. (1990) The diary as a formative teaching and learning aid incorporating means of evaluation and re-negotiation of clinical learning objectives. *Nurse Educator Today*, Vol. 10, pp. 228–32.

Mahrer, A.L. (1989) A case of fundamentally different existential-humanistic psychologies. *Journal of Humanistic Psychology*, 29 (2): 249–61.

Maslow, A.H. (1972) *Motivation and Personality*, 2nd edn. New York, Harper and Row.

Maslow, A.H. (1950) *Self-Actualising People: A Study of Psychological Health*. Personality Symposia I. New York, Grune and Stratton.

Masson, J. (1988) *Against Therapy*. London, Fontana/Collins.

May, R. (1989) Answer to Ken Wilber and John Rowan. *Journal of Humanistic Psychology*, 29 (2): 244–8.

May, T. (1993) *Social Research: Issues, Methods and Processes*. Milton Keynes, Open University Press.

McCaugherty, D. (1991) The use of a teaching model to promote reflection and the experiential integration of theory and practice in first-year student nurses: an action research study. *Journal of Advanced Nursing*, 16: 534–43.

McLeod, J. (1998) *An Introduction to Counselling*. Milton Keynes, Open University Press.

Mezirow, J. (1981) A critical theory of adult learning and education. *Adult Education*, 32 (1): 3–24.

Miles, R. (1987) Experiential learning in the classroom. In P. Allan and M. Jolley (eds), *The Curriculum in Nursing Education*. London, Croom Helm.

Miller, F. (1991) Using Roy's model in a special hospital. *Nursing Times*, 5 (12): 29–32.

Miller, R. and Bor, R. (1992) Counselling in terminal care. *Nursing Times*, 6 (26): 52–5.

Miller, R., Goldman, K. and Ormanese, M. (1993) Bereavement counselling in HIV disease. *Nursing Standard*, 7 (39): 48–51.

Mok, J. (1989) Babies of HIV infected women in Edinburgh, *Midwifery*, 5: 17–20.

Moreno, J.L. (1959) *Psychodrama*, Vol. 2. Beacon, NY, Beacon House Press.

Moreno, J.L. (1969) *Psychodrama*, Vol. 3. Beacon, NY, Beacon House Press.

Moreno, J.L. (1977) *Psychodrama*, Vol. 1, 4th edn. Beacon, NY, Beacon House Press.

Morrison, P. (1989) Nursing and caring: a personal construct theory study of some nurses' self-perceptions. *Journal of Advanced Nursing*, 14: 421–6.

Morrison, P. and Burnard, P. (1989) Students' and trained nurses' perceptions of their own interpersonal skills: a report and comparison. *Journal of Advanced Nursing*, 14: 321–9.

Moustakas, C. (1984) *Finding Yourself, Finding Others*. Englewood Cliffs, NJ, Prentice Hall.

Munro-Faure, L., Munro-Faure, M. and Bones, E. (1993) *Achieving Quality Standards*. London, Pitman

Murphy, K. and Atkins, S. (1994) Reflection with a practice-led curriculum. In A.M. Palmer, S. Burns and C. Bulman (eds), *Reflective Practice in Nursing: The Growth of the Professional Practitioner*. London, Blackwell.

Musashi, M. (1645) *A Book of Five Rings* (translated by Victor Harris, 1974). London, Allison and Busby.

Nelson-Jones, R. (1981) *The Theory and Practice of Counselling Psychology*. London, Holt Rinehart and Winston.

O'Brien, M.E. (1982) The need for spiritual integrity. In H. Yura and W.B. Walsh (eds), *Human Needs 2 and the Nursing Process*. Norwalk, CT, Appleton–Century–Crofts.

Ornstein, R.E. (1975) *The Psychology of Consciousness*. Harmondsworth, Penguin.

Palmer, A., Burns, S. and Bulman, C. (eds) (1994) *Reflective Practice in Nursing: The Growth of the Professional Practitioner*. Oxford, Blackwell.

Pedersen, P. (1994) Multicultural counselling. In R.W. Brislin and T. Yoshida (eds), *Improving Intercultural Modules for Cross-cultural Training Programs*. Newbury Park, CA, Sage.

Peters, R.S. (1969) *Ethics and Education*. London, Allen and Unwin.

Peters, R.S. (1972) Education as initiation. In R.D. Archambault (ed.), *Philosophical Analysis and Education*. London, Routledge and Kegan Paul.

Peterson, E. (1985) The physical … the spiritual … Can you meet all of your patients needs? *Journal of Gerontological Nursing*, 11 (10): 23–7.

Pfeiffer, J.W. and Jones, J.E. (1974) *A Handbook of Structured Experiences for Human Relations Training*. La Jolla, CA: University Associates.

Polanyi, M. (1957) *Personal Knowledge* Chicago, University of Chicago Press.

Postman, N. and Weingartner, C. (1971) *Teaching as a Subversive Activity*. Harmondsworth, Penguin.

Powell, J.H. (1989) The reflective practitioner in nursing. *Journal of Advanced Nursing*, 14: 824–32.

Pring, R. (1976) *Knowledge and Schooling*. London, Open Books.

Reason, P. and Rowan, J. (1981) *Human Inquiry: A Sourcebook of New Paradigm Research*. Chichester, Wiley.

Reich, W. (1949) *Character Analysis*. New York, Simon and Schuster.

Reid, B. (1993) 'But we're doing it already!' Exploring a response to the concept of Reflective Practice in order to improve its facilitation. *Nurse Education Today*, 13: 305–9.

Reyner, J.H. (1984) *The Gurdjieff Inheritance*. Wellingborough, Turnstone Press.

Rhinehart, L. (1971/1999) *The Dice Man*. London, Harper Collins.

Rogers, C.R. (1952) *Client-Centered Therapy*. London, Constable.

Rogers, C.R. (1967) *On Becoming a Person*. London, Constable.

Rogers, C.R. (1983) *Freedom to Learn for the Eighties*. Columbus, OH, Merrill.

Rolf, I. (1973) *Structural Integration*. New York, Viking Press.

Roth A. and Fonagy, P. (1996) *What Works for Whom? A Critical Review of Psychotherapy Research*. London: Guilford Press.

Rowan, J. (1988) *Ordinary Ecstasy: Humanistic Psychology in Action*. London, Routledge.

Rowan, J. (1989a) The Self: one or many? *The Psychologist: Bulletin of the British Psychological Society*, 7: 279–81.

Rowan, J. (1989b) Two humanistic psychologies or one? *Journal of Humanistic Psychology*, 29 (2): 224–9.

Rowland. N., Bower, P., Mellor-Clark, J. *et al.* (2001) *Counselling for Depression in Primary Care* (Cochrane Review). *The Cochrane Library*, Issue 2. Oxford: Update Software.

Rowntree, D. (1977) *Assessing Students: How Shall We Know Them?* London, Harper and Row.

Ryle, G. (1949) *The Concept of Mind*. Harmondsworth, Peregrine.

Sapsford, R. and Abbott, P. (1992) *Research Methods for Nursing and the Caring Professionals*. Buckingham, Open University Press.

Sartre, J-P. (1956) *Being and Nothingness*. New York, Philosophical Library.

Sartre, J-P. (1964) *Words*. Harmondsworth, Penguin.

Sartre, J-P. (1965) *Nausea*. Harmondsworth, Penguin.

Sartre, J-P. (1973) *Humanism and Existentialism*. London, Methuen.

Sathe, V. (1983) Implications of corporate culture. A manager's guide to action. *Organizational Dynamics*, 12: 5–23.

Saylor, C.R. (1990) Reflection and professional education: art, science and competency. *Nurse Educator*, 15 (2): 8–11.

Schulman, E.D. (1982) *Intervention in Human Services: A Guide to Skills and Knowledge*, 3rd edn. St Louis, MI and Toronto, C.V. Mosby.

Searle, J.R. (1983) *Intentionality: An Essay in Philosophy of Mind*. Cambridge, Cambridge University Press.

Sedgwick, P. (1982) *Psychopolitics*. London, Pluto Press.

Seligman, M. (1995) The effectiveness of psychotherapy: the consumer reports study. *American Psychologist*, 50: 965–74.

Shaffer, J.B.P. (1978) *Humanistic Psychology*. Englewood Cliffs, NJ, Prentice Hall.

Shon, D. (1983) *The Reflective Practitioner: How Professionals Think in Action.* Temple Smith, London.

Shor, I. (1980) *Critical Teaching and Everyday Life.* Boston, MA, South End Press.

Sibbald, B., Ward, E. and King, M. (2000) Randomised controlled trial of non-directive counselling, cognitive-behaviour therapy and usual general practitioner care in the management of depression as well as mixed anxiety and depression in primary care. *Health Technology Assessment,* 4: 19.

Simpson, S., Corney, R., Fitzgerald, P. *et al.* (2000) A randomised controlled trial to evaluate the effectiveness and cost-effectiveness of counselling patients with chronic depression. *Health Technology Assessment,* 4: 36.

Singer, P.(1980) *Marx.* Oxford, Oxford University Press.

Smoyak, A.S. and Rouslin, S. (1982) *A Collection of Classics in Psychiatric Nursing Literature.* Thorofare, NJ, Slack.

Soeken, K. and Carson, V. (1986) Study measures of nurses' attitudes about providing spiritual care. *Health Progress,* April, pp. 52–5.

Spinelli, E. (1989) *The Interpreted World: An Introduction to Phenomenological Psychology.* London, Sage.

Steinbeck, J. (1961) *The Winter of Our Discontent.* London, Heinemann.

Stein-Parbury, J. (1993) *Patient and Person: Developing Interpersonal Skills in Nursing.* Edinburgh, Churchill Livingstone.

Stevens, J.O. (1971) *Awareness: Exploring, Experimenting, Experiencing.* Moab, Utah, Real People Press.

Tomlinson, A. (1985) The use of experiential methods in teaching interpersonal skills to nurses. In C.M. Kagan (ed.), *Interpersonal Skills in Nursing: Research and Applications.* London, Croom Helm.

Totton, N. and Edmonston, E. (1984) *Reichian Growth Work: Melting Blocks to Life and Love.* Bridgeport, Prism Press.

Tschudin, V. (1991) *Counselling Skills for Nurses,* 3rd edn. London, Ballière Tindall.

Tuckman, B.W. (1965) Developmental sequences in small groups. *Psychological Bulletin,* 63 (6): 384–99.

Vonnegut, K. (1968) *Mother Night.* London, Cape.

Walker, D.S. (1987) *Using Groups to Help People.* London, Routledge.

Ward, E., King, M., Lloyd, M. *et al.* (2000) Randomised controlled trial of non-directive counselling, cognitive-behaviour therapy and usual GP care for patients with depression. I: Clinical effectiveness. *British Medical Journal,* 321: 1383–8.

Weil, S. (1950/1967) *Waiting on God.* Glasgow, Collins.

Weil, S.W. and McGill, I. (eds) (1989) *Making Sense of Experiential Learning: Diversity in Theory and Practice.* Milton Keynes, Open University Press.

Whitehead, A.N. (1932) *The Aims of Education.* London, Benn.

Wilber, K. (1989) Two humanistic psychologies or one? A response. *Journal of Humanistic Psychology,* 29 (2): 230–43.

Wilkinson, R. (2000) Nishida and Satayana on Goethe: an essay in comparative aesthetics. *Journal of Comparative Literature and Aesthetics,* XXIII (1–2).

Wilson. C. (1965) *Beyond the Outsider: A Philosophy of the Future.* London, Pan.

Wirth, J. (1979) *John Dewey as Educator.* New York, Robert Krieger.

Wittgenstein, L. (1922/1961) *Tractatus Logico-Philosophicus.* London, Routledge and Kegan Paul.

Wlodkowski, J. (1985) *Enhancing Adult Motivation to Learn.* San Francisco, Jossey Bass.

Wood, D. (1971) Strategies. In S. and R. Godlovitch and J. Harris (eds), *Animals, Men and Mortals*. London, Gollancz.

Woolfolk, R.L. and Sass, L.A. (1989) Behaviourism and existentialism revisted. *Journal of Humanistic Psychology*, 28 (1): 108–19.

Wyatt, P. (1993) The role of the nurse in counselling the terminally ill patient. *British Journal of Nursing*, 2 (14): 701–5.

Yardley, K. & Honess, T. (1987) (Eds.). *Self and Identity: Psychosocial perspectives*. Chichester: John Wiley.

Zweig, F. (1965) The Quest for Fellowship. London, Heinemann.

Bibliography

Abrahams, P. (1984) Evaluating soft findings: some problems of measuring informal care. *Research, Policy and Planning*, 2 (2): 1–8.

Adler, R.B., Rosenfield, L.B. and Towne, N. (1983) *Interplay: The Process of Interpersonal Communication*. London, Holt, Rinehart and Winston.

Allcock, N. (1992) Teaching the skills of assessment through the use of an experiential workshop. *Nurse Education Today*, 12 (4), 287–92.

Ashworth, P.D. and Longmate, M.A. (1993) Theory and practice: beyond the dichotomy. *Nurse Education Today*, 13 (5): 321–7.

Ashworth, P.D., Giorgi, A. and de Koning, A.J.J. (eds) (1986) Qualitative research in psychology. *Proceedings of the International Association for Qualitative Research, Duquesne, IO*

Atkins, S., Murphy, K. (1993) Critical thinking: a foundation for consumer-focused care. *Journal of Continuing Education in Nursing*, 18 (8): 1188–92.

Auerbach, K.G. (1991) Assisting the employed breastfeeding mother. *Breastfeeding Review*, 2 (4): 158–66.

Bailey, R. and Clarke, M (1989) *Stress and Coping in Nursing*. London, Chapman and Hall.

Barber, P. and Norman, I. (1987) Social skills in supervision. *Nursing Times*, 83: 14 January, pp. 56–7.

Bayntun, Lees D. (1993) Setting the scene for experiential learning. *Nursing Standard*, 7 (36): 28–30.

Benson, H. (1976) *The Relaxation Response*. London, Collins.

Berg, B.L. (1989) *Qualitative Research Methods for the Social Sciences*. Allyn and Bacon, New York.

Bodley, D.E. (1992) Clinical supervision in psychiatric nursing: using the process record. *Nurse Education Today*, 12: 148–55.

Boot, D., Gillies, P., Fenelon, J., Reubin, R., Wilkins, M. and Gray, P. (1994) Evaluation of the short-term impact of counseling in general practice. *Patient Education and Counselling*, 24: 79–89.

Bor, R. and Watts, M. (1993) Talking to patients about sexual matters. *British Journal of Nursing*, 2 (13): 657–61.

Boud, D., Keogh, R. and Walker, D. (1985) *Reflection: Turning Experience into Learning*. London, Kogan Page.

Bower, P. and King, M. (2000) Randomised controlled trials and the evaluation of psychological therapy. In N. Rowland and S. Goss (eds), *Evidence-based Counselling and Psychological Therapies*. London, Routledge, pp. 79–110.

Bracken, E. and Davis, J. (1989) The implications of mentorship in nursing career development. *Senior Nurse*, 9: 15–16.

Brandon, D. (1991) Counselling mentally ill people. *Nursing Standard*, 6 (7): 32–3.

Brookfield, S. (1993) On impostorship, cultural suicide and other dangers: how nurses learn critical thinking. *Journal of Continuing Education in Nursing*, 24 (5): 197–205.

Bryman, A. (1988) *Quantity and Quality in Social Research*. London, Unwin Hyman.

Buchan, R. (1991) An integrated model of counselling. *Senior Nurse*, 11 (4): 32–3.

Buckroyd, J. and Smith, E. (1990) Learning to help ... teaching counselling. *Nursing Times*, 86 (35): pp. 54–7.

Burnard, P. (1987) Towards an epistemological basis for experiential learning. *Journal of Advanced Nursing*, 12: 289–193.

Burnard, P. (1988) Preventing burnout. *Journal of District Nursing*, 7 (5): 9–10.

Burnard, P. (1990) Learning from Experience: Nurse Tutors' and Student Nurses' Perceptions of Experiential Learning. Unpublished PhD Thesis, University of Wales.

Burnard, P. (1990) *Learning Human Skills: An Experiential Guide for Nurses*, 2nd edn. Oxford, Heinemann.

Burnard, P. (1992) *Experiential Learning in Action*. Aldershot, Avebury.

Burnard, P. and Morrison, P. (1991) Client-centred counselling: a study of nurses' attitudes, *Nurse Education Today*, 11: 104–9.

Burnard, P. and Morrison, P. (1991) Nurses' interpersonal skills: a study of nurses' perceptions, *Nurse Education Today*, 11 (1): 24–9.

Byrne, S. (1991) Counselling – and essential nursing skill. *World of Irish Nursing*, 20 (4): 26–7.

Cameron, B.L. and Mitchell, A.M. (1993) Reflective peer journals: developing authentic nurses. *Journal of Advanced Nursing*, 18 (2): 290–17.

Carpio, B.A. and Majumdar, B. (1993) Experiential learning: an approach to transcultural education for nursing. *Journal of Transcultural Nursing*, 4 (2): 4–11.

Carty, E.M., Conine, T.A. and Hall, L. (1990) Comprehensive health promotion for the pregnant woman who is disabled: the role of the midwife. *Journal of Nurse Midwifery*, 353: 133–42.

Chambless, D. and Hollon, S. (1998) Defining empirically supported therapies. *Journal of Consulting and Clinical Psychology*, 66: 7–18.

Chateauvert, M., Duffie, A. and Gilmore, N. (1991) Human immunodeficiency virus antibody testing: counselling guidelines from the Canadian Medical Association. *Patient Education and Counselling*, 18 (1): 35–49.

Cheek, J., Gibson, T. and Heartfield, M. (1993) Holism, care and nursing: points of reflection during the evolution of a philosophy of nursing statement. *Contemporary Nurse: A Journal for the Australian Nursing Profession*, 2 (2): 68–72

Clare, J. (1993) A challenge to the rhetoric of emancipation: recreating a professional culture, *Journal of Advanced Nursing*, 18(7): 1033–8.

Clark, J.M., Hopper, L. and Jesson, A. (1991) Communication skills: progression to counselling. *Nursing Times*, 87 (8): 41–3.

Clarke, C. and Watson, D. (1991) Informal carers of the dementing elderly: a study of relationships. *Nursing Practice*, 4 (4), pp. 17–21.

Clarke, J.M., Hopper, L. and Jesson, A. (1991) Communication skills: progression to counselling. *Nursing Times*, 87 (8): 41–3.

Clarke, L. (1989) Intervention and certainty in counselling literature: Part 1, *Senior Nurse*, 9 (4): 18–19.

Clarke, M. (1986) Action and reflection: practice and theory in nursing, *Journal of Advanced Nursing*, 11: 3–11.

Claus, K.E. and Bailey, J.T. (1980) *Living with Stress and Promoting Wellbeing: A Handbook for Nurses*. St Louis, MI, C.V. Mosby.

Clift, I. and Magee, T. (1992) Developing a new counselling course, *Nursing Standard*, 6 (18), 34–6

Cook, S.W. and Selltiz, C. (1973) A multiple indicator approach to attitudinal measurement. In N. Warne and M. Jahoda (eds), *Attitudes*, 2nd edn. Penguin, Harmondsworth.

Costello, J. (1989) Learning from each other: peer teaching and learning in student nurse training. *Nurse Education Today*, 9: 203–6.

Crandall, S. (1993) How expert clinical educators teach what they know, *Journal of Continuing Education in the Health Professions*, 13 (1): 85–98.

Crowne, D.P. and Marlowe, D. (1964) *The Approval Motive*. New York, Wiley.

Curtis, T. and Kibler, S. (1990) Counselling in cancer care. *Nursing Times*, 86 (51): 25–7.

Cutcliffe, J.R. and Cassedy, P. (1999) The development of empathy in students on a short, skills based counselling course: a pilot study. *Nurse Education Today*, 19 (3): 250–7.

Darbyshire, P. (1993) In the hall of mirrors . . . reflective practice. *Nursing Times*, 89 (49): 26–9.

Dass, R. (1977) *The Only Dance There Is*. New York, Anchor Press.

Davies, J.M. (1991) A behavioural model for counselling the nursing mother. *Breastfeeding Review*, 2 (4), pp. 154–7.

Davis, B.D. (1981) *Social Skills in Nursing*. In M. Argyle (ed.), *Social Skills and Health*. London, Methuen.

Davison, J. (1992) Approach with care . . . individual or group counselling. *Nursing Times*, 88 (8), pp. 38–9.

Denton, P.L. (1992) Teaching interpersonal skills with videotape to chronically ill psychiatric clients, *Occupational Therapy in Mental Health*, 2 (4): 17–34.

Derogatis, H. (1993) A different reflection . . . growing up with cerebral palsy. *Nursing Outlook*, 41 (5): 235–7.

Dewing, J. (1990) Reflective practice . . . within primacy nursing from individual and group viewpoints, *Senior Nurse*, 10 (10): 26–8.

Dimmock, B. (1992) A child of our own . . . frequency and intensity of problems about pregnancy and young children in stepfamilies. *Health Visitor*, 65 (10): 368–70.

Dives, D.M. (1993) An assessment of the value of health education in the prevention of childhood asthma. *Journal of Advanced Nursing*, 18 (3): 354–63.

Docking, S. (1994) Accredited learning – the assessment procedure: how to complete the assessment for the reflective practice module. *Professional Nurse*, 9 (4): 244 6.

Donovan, J. (1990) The concept and role of mentor. *Nurse Education Today*, 10: 294–8.

Doust, M. (1991) Student nurses and counselling services. Nursing Standard, 5 (15/16): 35–7.

Dux, C.M. (1989) An investigation into whether nurse teachers take into account the individual learning styles of the students when formulating teaching strategies. *Nurse Education Today*, 9: 186–91.

Ellis, C. (1993) Incorporating the affective domain into staff development programs. *Journal of Nursing Staff Development*, 9 (3): 127–30.

ENB (1982) *Syllabus of Training: Professional Register–Part 3: Registered Mental Nurse*. London, English National Board for Nursing, Midwifery and Health Visiting.

English, K., Rojeski, T. and Branham, K. (2000) Acquiring counseling skills in mid-career: outcomes of a distance education course for practicing audiologists. *Journal of the American Academy of Audiology*, 11 (2): 84–90.

Farrington, A. (1993) Intuition and expert clinical practice in nursing. *British Journal of Nursing*, 2 (4): 228–9.

Fink, A. and Kosecoff, J. (1985) *How to Conduct Surveys: A Step-By-Step Guide.* Beverly Hills, CA, Sage.

Firth, S. (1999 Counseling model: creating a healing environment in hospitals. *Patient Education and Counseling*, 36 (1): 81–9.

French, P. and Cross, D. (1992) An interpersonal epistemological curriculum model for nurse education. *Journal of Advanced Nursing*, 17 (1): 83–9.

Friedli, K., King, M. and Lloyd, M. (2000) The economics of employing a counsellor in general practice: analysis of data from a randomised controlled trial. *British Journal of General Practice*. 50: 276–83.

Frisz, R.H. (1999) Multicultural peer counseling: counselling the multicultural student. *Journal of Adolescence*, 22 (4): 515–26.

Gamel, C. and Davis, B.D. and Hengeveld, M. (1993) Nurses' provision of teaching and counselling on sexuality: review of the literature. *Journal of Advanced Nursing*, 18 (8): 1219–27.

Garrett, R. (1983) The power of action learning. In M. Pedlar (ed.), *Action Learning in Practice*. Aldershot, Gower.

Gaston, S. (1991) Sampling: an experiential learning activity. *Nurse Educator* 16 (5): 4, 12.

Gilbey, V. (1990) Screening and counselling clinic evaluation project. *Canadian Journal of Nursing Research*, 22 (3): 23–38.

Gillam, T. (1993) Representational systems in counselling. *Nursing Standard*, 8 (10): 25–7.

Ginsburg, C. (1984) Towards a somatic understanding of self. *Journal of Humanistic Psychology*, 24 (2): 66–92.

Glaser, B.G. and Strauss, A.L. (1967) *The Discovery of Grounded Theory*. New York, Aldine.

Gould, D. (1990) Empathy: a review of the literature with suggestions for an alternative research strategy. *Journal of Advanced Nursing*, 15 (10): 1167–74.

Gray, G. and Pratt, T. (1993) *Towards a Discipline of Nursing*. Edinburgh, Churchill Livingstone.

Greenwood, J. (1993) Reflective practice: a critique of the work of Argyris and Schon. *Journal of Advanced Nursing*, 18 (8): 1183–7.

Greenwood, J. (1993) Some considerations concerning practice and feedback in nursing education. *Journal of Advanced Nursing*, 18 (12): 1999–2000.

Guinn, C.A. (1992) Experiential learning: a 'real-world' introduction for baccalaureate nursing students. *Nurse Educator*, 17 (3): 31, 36.

Harvey, T.L. and Vaughan, J. (1990) Student nurse attitudes towards different teaching/learning methods. *Nurse Education Today*, 10: 181–5.

Hasler, K. (1993) Bereavement counselling. *Nursing Standard*, 7 (40): 31–6.

Hewitt, J. (1978) *Meditation*. Sevenoaks, Hodder and Stoughton.

Humberman, A.M. and Miles, M. (1994) *Data Management and Analysis Methods.* In N.K. Denzin and Y.S. Lincoln (eds), *Handbook of Qualitative Research.* Thousand Oaks, CA, Sage.

Iwasiw, C.L. and Sleightholm-Cairns, B. (1990) Clinical conferences – the key to successful experiential learning. *Nurse Education Today*, 10: 260–5.

Jacobson, N. and Christensen, A. (1996) Studying the effectiveness of psychotherapy: how well can clinical trials do the job? *American Psychologist*, 51: 1031–9.

James, C.R. and Clarke, B.A. (1994) Reflective practice in nursing: issues and implications for nurse education. *Nurse Education Today*, 14: 89–90.

Jarvis, P. (1987) *Adult Learning in the Social Context*. London, Croom Helm.

Jeavons, B. (1991) Developing counselling skills. *Nursing (London): The Journal of Clinical Practice Education and Management*, 4 (38): 28–9.

Jones, A. (1991) The path towards a common goal: structuring the counselling process. *Professional Nurse*, 6 (6): 302, 304–6.

Jones, A. (1992) Confronting the inevitable ... counselling ... a patient. *Nursing Standard*, 6 (46): 54–6.

Jones, A. (1993) A first step in effective communication: providing a supportive environment for counselling in hospital. *Professional Nurse*, 8 (8): 501–2, 502–5.

Jones, C. (1990) All you ever wanted to know about ... counselling. *Nursing Times*, pp. 55–8.

Jones, J. (1991) Therapeutic use of metaphor. *Nursing Standard*, 6 (11): 30–2.

Jukes, M. and O'Shea, K. (1998) Transcultural therapy. 2: Mental health and learning disabilities. *British Journal of Nursing*, 7 (20): 1268–72.

Kilty, J. (1978) *Self and Peer Assessment*. Guildford, Human Potential Research Project, University of Surrey.

Knight, J. (1992) The lecturer practitioner [*sic*]role: exploration and reflection. *Journal of Clinical Nursing*, 1 (2): 58–9.

Kramer, M.K. (1993) Concept clarification and critical thinking: integrated processes. *Journal of Nursing Education*, 32(9): 406–14.

Laitakari, J. (1998) How to develop one's counselling – demonstration of the use of single-case studies as a practical tool for evaluating the outcomes of counseling. *Patient Education and Counseling*, 33 (1 Suppl.): S39–46.

Laitakari, J. and Asikainen, T.M. (1998) How to promote physical activity through individual counselling – a proposal for a practical model of counseling on health-related physical activity. *Patient Education and Counseling*, 33 (1 Suppl.): S13–24.

Laschinger, H.K. and Tresolini C.P. (1999) An exploratory study of nursing and medical students health promotion counselling self-efficacy. *Nurse Education Today*, 19 (5): 408–18.

Lassman, S.K. (1999) Counselling training for complementary therapists: how much can it help the healing encounter? *Complementary Therapies in Medicine*, 7 (3): 186–8.

Lauder, W. (1994) Beyond reflection: practical wisdom and the practical syllogism. *Nurse Education Today*, 14: 91–98.

Le Shan, L. (1974) *How to Meditate*. Wellingborough, Turnstone Press.

Levin, B. (1998) Grief counseling. *American Journal of Nursing*, 98 (5): 69–72.

Lewin, K. (1952) *Field Theory and Social Change*. London, Tavistock.

Lewis, D. (1998) Clinical supervision for nurse lecturers. *Nursing Standard*, 12 (29): 40–3.

Lewis, F.M. and Zahlis, E.H. (1997) The nurse as coach: a conceptual framework for clinical practice. *Oncology Nursing Forum*, 24 (10):1695–702.

Lindsey, E. and Attridge, C. (1989) Staff nurses' perceptions of support in an acute care workplace. *Canadian Journal of Nursing Research*, 21 (2): pp. 15–25.

Luft, J. (1984) *Group Processes: An Introduction to Group Dynamics*, 2nd edn. San Francisco, Mayfield.

Macleod Clark, J. and Faulkner, A. (1987) Communication skills teaching in nurse education. In B.D. Davis (ed.), *Nursing Education: Research and Developments*. London, Croom Helm.

Mahony, C. (1999) You want to be a ... counsellor. *Nursing Times*, 95 (14): 34–5.

Mander, R. (1992) See how they learn: experience as the basis of practice. *Nurse Education Today*, 121: 3–10.

Marita, P., Leena, L. and Tarja, K. (1999) Nurses' self-reflection via videotaping to improve communication skills in health counseling. *Patient Education and Counseling*, 36 (1): 3–11.

Marshfield, G. (1985) Issues Arising from Teaching Interpersonal Skills in General Nurse Training. In C. Kagan (ed.), *Interpersonal Skills in Nursing: Research and Applications*. London, Croom Helm.

Marte, A.L. (1991) Experiential learning strategies for promoting positive staff attitudes toward the elderly. *Journal of Continuing Education in Nursing*, 22 (2): 73–7.

Maslach, C. (1981) *Burnout: the Cost of Caring*. Englewood Cliffs, NJ, Prentice Hall.

Mason, P. (1992) Allowing for loss – bereavement counselling. *Nursing Times*, 88 (2): 14–15.

McBride, C.M. and Rimer, B.K. (1999) Using the telephone to improve health behavior and health service delivery. Patient Education and Counseling, 1: 3–18.

McIntee, J. and Firth, H. (1984) How to beat the burnout. *Health and Social Services Journal*, 9 February, pp. 166–8.

McMillan, I. (1991) A listening ear … telephone counselling, *Nursing Times*, 87 (6): 30–1.

McWilliams, S. (1991) Affective changes following severe head injury as perceived by patients and relatives. *British Journal of Occupational Therapy*, 54 (7): 246–8.

Melby, V. (1992) Counselling of patients with HIV related diseases: what is the role of the nurse?, *Journal of Clinical Nursing*, 1 (1): 39–45.

Meyeroff, M. (1972) On Caring. New York, Harper and Row.

Moore, E.R., Bianchi-Gray, M. and Stephens, P. (1992) A Community Hospital-based breastfeeding counselling service. *Breastfeeding Review*, 2 (6): 264–70.

Morrison, P. (1992) *Professional Caring in Practice: A Psychological Analysis*. Aldershot, Avebury.

Morrison, P., Burnard, P. and Hackett, P. (1991) A smallest space analysis of nurses' perceptions of their interpersonal skills. *Counselling Psychology Quarterly*, 4 (2/3): 119–25.

Neale, J. (1993) Emotional aspects of HIV. *Physiotherapy*, 79 (3): 173–7.

Newell, R. (1992) Anxiety, accuracy and reflection: the limits of professional development. *Journal of Advanced Nursing*, 17 (11): 1326–33.

Nkowane, A.M. (1993) Breaking the silence: the need for counselling of HIV/AIDS patients. *International Nursing Review*, 40 (1): 17–20, 24.

Noell, J. and Glasgow, R.E. (1999) Interactive technology applications for behavioral counseling: issues and opportunities for health care settings. *American Journal of Preventive Medicine*, 17 (4): 269–74.

Nupponen, R. (1998) What is counseling all about – basics in the counseling of health-related physical activity. *Patient Education and Counseling*, 33 (1 Suppl): S61–7.

O'Kell, S.P. (1988) A study of the relationship between learning style, readiness for self-directed learning and teaching preference of learner nurses in one health district. *Nurse Education Today*, 8: 197–204.

Palmer, R. and Pope, C. (1984) *Brain Train: Studying for Success*. London, Spon.

Paunonen, M. (1991) Testing a model for counsellor training in three public health care organizations. *Nurse Education Today*, 11 (4): 270–7.

Perls, F. (1969) *Ego, Hunger and Aggression*. New York, Random House.

Perls, F. (1969) *Gestalt Therapy Verbatim*. Lafayette, CA, Real People Press.

Petty, J. (1962) *Apples of Gold*. New York, Walker and Co.

Phillips, J. (1993) Counselling and the nurse. *British Journal of Theatre Nursing*, 2 (10): 13.

Pierce, J.C. (1982) *The Bond of Power: Meditation and Wholeness*. London, Routledge.

Pope, V.T. and Kline, W.B. (1999) The personal characteristics of effective counselors: what 10 experts think. *Psychological Reports*, 84 (3 Pt 2): 1339–44.

Progoff, I. (1985) *The Dynamics of Hope*. New York, Dialogue House Library.

Pulsford, D. (1993) Reducing the threat: an experiential exercise to introduce role play to student nurses. *Nurse Education Today*, 13 (2): 145–8.

Pulsford, D. (1993) The reluctant participant in experiential learning. *Nurse Education Today*, 13 (2): 139–44.

Quinsland, L.K. and Van Ginkel, A. (1984) How to process experience. *Journal of Experiential Education*, 7 (2): 8–13.

Raichura, L. (1987) Learning by doing. *Nursing Times*, 83 (13): 59–61.

Ramos, M.C. (1992) The nurse–patient relationship: theme and variations. *Journal of Advanced Nursing*, 17: 496–506.

Reid, W. and Long, A. (1993) The role of the nurse providing therapeutic care for the suicidal patient. *Journal of Advanced Nursing*, 18: 1369–76.

Reilly, D.E. and Oermann, M.II. (1985) *The Clinical Field: Its Use in Nursing Education*. Norwalk, CT, Appleton–Century–Crofts.

Reynolds, W. (1985) Issues arising from teaching interpersonal skills in psychiatric nurse training. In C. Kagan (ed.), *Interpersonal Skills in Nursing. Research and Applications*. London, Croom Helm.

Reynolds, W. and Cormack, D. (1987) Teaching psychiatric nursing: interpersonal skills. In B. Davis (ed.), *Nurse Education: Research and Developments*. London, Croom Helm.

Ricketts, T. (1993) Therapist self-disclosure in behavioural psychotherapy. *British Journal of Nursing*, 2 (13): 667–71.

Robertson, A. (1999) The power of the group. *Practising Midwife*, 2 (4): 16–17.

Robotham, A. (1992) The use of credit and experiential learning in nurse education. Exciting opportunities for student and tutor alike. *Nurse Education Today*, 11 (6): 448–53.

Rogers, C.R. (1972) The process of the basic encounter group. In R. Dietrich and H. Dye (eds), *Group Procedures: Purposes, Processes and Outcomes*. Boston, MA, Houghton Mifflin.

Rogers, C.R. (1985) Towards a more human science of the person. *Journal of Humanistic Psychology*, 25: 7–24.

Rogers, C.R. and Stevens, B. (1967) *Person to Person: The Problem of Being Human*. Lafayette, CA, Real People Press.

Rolfe, G. (1990) The assessment of therapeutic attitudes in the psychiatric setting. *Journal of Advanced Nursing*, 15 (5): 564–70.

Rolfe, G. (1990) The role of clinical supervision in the education of student psychiatric nurses: a theoretical approach. *Nurse Education Today*, 10 (3): 193–7.

Rolfe, G. (1993) Closing the theory practice gap: a model of nursing praxis, *Journal of Clinical Nursing*, 2 (2): 89–93.

Rugg, D.L. *et al.* (1992) Evaluating the CDC programme for HIV counselling and testing. *International Nursing Review*, 39 (5): 157–60.

Sankar, S. (1987) Teaching psychiatric nursing: curriculum development for the 1982.

Syllabus. In B.D. Davis (ed.), *Nurse Education: Research and Developments*. London, Croom Helm.

Sarantakos, S. (1993) *Social Research*. London, Macmillan.

Savage, P. (1997 Philosophical counselling. *Nursing Ethics*, 4(1): 39–48.

Schutz, W. (1973) *Elements of Encounter*. New York, Irvington.

Silverman, D. (1985) *Qualitative Methodology and Sociology*. Aldershot, Gower.

Simon, S.B., Howe, L.W. and Kirshenbaum, H. (1978) *Values Clarification*, rev. edn. New York, A. and W. Visual Library.

Smith, P.B. (1980) *Group Processes and Personal Change*. London, Harper and Row.

Smith, Stevie (1975) *Selected Poems*. Harmondsworth, Penguin.

Snyder, M. (1993) Critical thinking: a foundation for consumer-focused care. *Journal of Continuing Education in Nursing*, 24 (5): 206–10.

Soohbany, M.S. (1999) Counselling as part of the nursing fabric: where is the evidence? A phenomenological study using 'reflection on actions' as a tool for framing the 'lived counselling experiences of nurses'. *Nurse Education Today*, 9 (1): 35–40.

Speck, P. (1992) Managing the boundaries ... using our counselling skills to help a colleague or a student can create more problems. *Nursing Times*, 88 (32): 22.

Spolin, V. (1963) *Improvisations for the Theatre*. Evanston, IL, Northwestern University Press.

Steel, S.M. and Harmon, V.M. (1983) *Values Clarification in Nursing*, 2nd edn. Norwalk, CT, Appleton–Century–Crofts.

Tart, C. (ed.) (1969) *Altered States of Consciousness*. New York, Wiley.

Thorne, B. and Dryden, W. (1993) *Counselling: Interdisciplinary Perspectives*. Buckingham: Open University Press.

Thorne, P. (1991) Assessment of prior experiential learning. *Nursing Standard*, 6 (10): 32–4.

Toropainen, E. and Rinne, M. (1998) What are groups all about? Basic principles of group work for health-related physical activity. *Patient Education and Counseling*, 3 (1 Suppl): S105–9.

Vauderslott, J. (1992) A supportive therapy that undermines violence: counselling to prevent ward violence. *Professional Nurse*, 7 (7): 427–8, 430.

Vaughan, F. (1984) Discovering transpersonal identity. *Journal of Humanistic Psychology*, 25 (3): 13–38.

Victor, C., Jefferies, S. and Sherr, L. (1993) Improving counselling skills: training in obstetric and paediatric HIV and AIDS. *Professional Care of Mother and Child*, 3 (4): 97–100.

Walsh, K.K., VandenBosch, T.M. and Boehm, S. (1989) Modelling and role modelling: integrating nursing theory and practice. *Journal of Advanced Nursing*, 14: 755–61.

Wilber, K. (1981) *Up From Eden: A Transpersonal View of Human Evolution*. London, Routledge and Kegan Paul.

Wilkins, H. (1993) Transcultural nursing: a selective review of the literature: 1985–1991. *Journal of Advanced Nursing*, 184: 602–12.

Wilshaw, G. (1997) Integration of therapeutic approaches: a new direction for mental health nurses? *Journal of Advanced Nursing*, 26 (1): 15–19.

Winship, G. and Hardy, S. (1999) Disentangling dynamics: group sensitivity and supervision. *Journal of Psychiatric and Mental Health Nursing*, 6 (4): 307–12.

Wituk, S., Shepherd, M.D., Slavich, S., Warren, M.L. and Meissen, G. (2000) A topography of self-help groups: an empirical analysis. *Social Work*, 45 (2): 157–65.

Wondrak, R. and Goble, J. (1992) An investigation into self, peer and tutor assessments of student psychiatric nurses written work assignments. *Nurse Education Today*, 12 (1): 61–4.

Wright, J. (1991) Counselling at the cultural interface: is getting back to roots enough? *Journal of Advanced Nursing*, 16 (1): 92–100.

Zahourek, R.P. (ed.) (1988) *Relaxation and Imagery: Tools for Therapeutic Communication and Intervention*. Philadelphia, Saunders.

Index